EATING THE LORD'S WAY

A STEP-BY-STEP GUIDE
TO LIVING
THE WORD OF WISDOM

BY

KAREN
HOPKINS

Eating the Lord's Way: A Step-by-Step Guide to Living the Word of Wisdom

GENESIS 1:29

And God said, Behold, I have given you every herb bearing seed, which is upon the face of all the earth, and every tree in the which is the fruit of a tree yielding seed; to you it shall be for meat.

Other Books by Karen Hopkins:

Shaman Priest

Down the Colorado

Sparrow Hawk

Up the Devil's Highway

Monster Slayer's Son

White Shell Woman's Promise

Sugar Cane

Isaiah and Me

CONTENTS

.

Recipes by Category page

Foil Dinner Fish

Skillet Scallops

Salmon with Spinach

Tuna on Cheesy Rice

179 LEGUMES

Black beans and rice

Black beans w corn, tomatoes

No Meat Chimichangas

Refried Bean Soup

Katie's Chili Beans

183 SALADS

Artichoke Avocado Salad

Beet and Potato Salad

Bean Salad

Broccoli Apple Salad

Cabbage Salad

Chopped Salad

Cucumber Salad

Fruit Salad

Chilean Onion Tomato Salad

Papaya Avocado Salad

189 SAUCES, SALSAS

Artichoke salsa

Cheese Sauce

Pico de Gallo

Spinach Dip

Terrific Tomato Sauce

Vinaigrette

White Sauce

Chilies & Queso Salsa

East Mayonnaise

Pesto Mayonnaise

Garlic Oil

Guacamole

194 SIDES

Garlic Spinach

Herbed New Potatoes

Mexican Brown Rice

Ratatouille

Sliced Baked Potatoes

Zucchini and Tomatoes

Zucchini au Gratin

198 SOUPS, STEWS

Acorn Soup

Black Bean Soup

Chunky Potato Soup

Portugal's Cabbage Soup

Lentil Veggie Soup

Minestrone Soup

Potato Green Chili Soup

Pumpkin Soup

Split Pea Soup

Vegetable Soup

Fresh Vegetable Soup

Tomato Basil Soup

206 VEGETARIAN ENTRES

Brazilian Empanadas

Broccoli Casserole

Broccoli Potato Sauté

Broccoli Empanadas

Brown Rice with Veggies

Calzone

Cheese Spinach Manicotti

Cheesy Enchiladas

Mexican Lasagna

Potato Apple Casserole

Stew

INTRODUCTION

Why another book on the Word of Wisdom?

There are lots of good reasons to study and follow the dietary advice found in the Word of Wisdom. But for me this book started with a conversation. Not too long ago I was talking to one of my sons about the wisdom in the Word of Wisdom. He asked me if I thought drinking coffee was immoral. I thought about it for just a minute before I answered, "No. Billions of good people all over the world drink coffee. Drinking coffee is not a moral choice; it's a health choice." And that simple question and answer changed to some degree the way I think about the Word of Wisdom.

What is the Word of Wisdom? It is our guideline to good health, but it is not a moral law. People can drink alcohol, smoke tobacco, drink coffee and tea and still be good and moral people (although we sometimes judge folks rather harshly for indulging in those unhealthy practices.) Removing the moral stigma and focusing on the Word of

Wisdom as a God-given guideline to a better, healthier life changes the way we think about the entire Word of Wisdom, the do's as well as the do not's, and it helps us focus on the positive as well as the negative health advice contained in this valuable revelation.

To fully live the Word of Wisdom it is not enough to simply avoid a few unhealthy substances. It's good to avoid those substances, there's no question about that, and health statistics bear out the benefits we receive. But why not take advantage of the whole Word of Wisdom and enjoy the good health the Lord intends us to have?

I have always been interested in health and nutrition. I took my first nutrition class at BYU back in 1969 or so. I remember wondering about some of the things that were taught in that course: for example, the teacher explained that weight gain was a simple matter of calorie intake. It didn't matter what types of food we ate; a calorie was a calorie and only by controlling or limiting the number of calories in our diet could we hope to control weight— except, she added, in a few rare cases of individuals with metabolic disorders. So, 1800 calories of Twinkies would have the same affect on my body as 1800 calories of carrot sticks? Hmmm?

I didn't buy it.

I didn't buy it then and I am happy to see that now to quote Mark Hyman, "Calories in, calories out is a completely disproven hypothesis." (1)

There are several ways to gain (or lose) weight. One is to eat too much or too little. It is possible to starve yourself, and it is possible to overeat. But by far the more common way to gain excess weight is to eat the wrong kinds of foods. Foods that affect insulin levels for instance, which in turn affect the metabolism, impact fat storage, weight gain, energy levels, and overall well-being. Hormonal or glandular imbalances can also affect weight and health, and so can stress. Cortisol, a hormone released in times of stress, can cause the body to store excess fat even for people on a very restricted diet. Imbalances or disruptions in the intestinal biome—all those friendly and not so friendly little bacteria, fungi and viruses that reside in and regulate our gut, can affect our health and weight. Our digestive system is so much more complicated than the plumbing in a sink, that the old calories in/calories out model simply doesn't work. Counting calories is not the key to good health or to a healthy body weight.

More important than the number of calories is the type of foods we eat and the effects those foods have on insulin and other hormones in our bodies. Weight is not the only thing affected by what we eat, but weight is in many ways an indication of whether our body is functioning properly. It is the types of foods we eat that form the foundation of our health, good or bad, and affect the functioning of the body's systems. It matters *what* we eat.

To enjoy optimal health it is important to give our body the foods it needs to function well, the foods that are right for us as humans. Figuring out what those foods are can be confusing. There is so much conflicting information out there, and making wise nutritional choices is the greatest single step we can take in maintaining or restoring good health, the health the Lord wants for us. So how do we decide what information to follow?

Back in that early nutrition class my teacher insisted that all forms of sugar were equal, that there was no difference between cane sugar in all its forms, corn syrup, honey, maple syrup, high fructose corn syrup and so on. In fact since all carbohydrates are broken down into glucose, she explained, it didn't matter what types of sugars OR carbs we ate. Still the skeptic, I knew I was going to have to look a little deeper if I hoped to find answers to what I thought constituted good nutrition and by extension good health. Unfortunately there is still a lot of misinformation and a lot we don't know when it comes to nutrition. But there is good information out there.

Now, many years after taking that first nutrition class, I have a grandson who is sucrose intolerant. He cannot eat sucrose in any form, whether as white sugar, brown sugar, or any of the other many names given to cane and beet sugar derivatives. He can't eat the sucrose used as a sweetener in ketchup or ice cream, in cakes, cookies, crackers, bread, soda, lemonade, spaghetti sauce, or so many other things. Sucrose is everywhere and sucrose makes him very ill, so ill that it almost ended his life before doctors identified the problem. But he can eat and digest without any problem honey, fructose, and even high fructose corn syrup. That's funny isn't it? I am not advocating for any of these sweeteners, but they are definitely NOT all the same. Yes, they all end up as glucose, but the path they take matters.

Let me repeat, while sweeteners aren't the healthiest diet choice (we'll talk about that later), they are definitely not all the same, and just because all carbs are eventually reduced to glucose doesn't mean they get there the same way. Our digestive system is more complex than that.

Eventually I began looking for a diet based on what the Word of Wisdom has to offer. After all, the Lord understands our bodies and knows the answers. But no program I encountered seemed complete. There are some "Word of Wisdom" diets that rely almost entirely on existing popular diet programs with very little adjustment for what the Word of Wisdom specifically says. Those diets may have worked well for some authors, but to me it felt like they were trying to fit the Word of Wisdom into a program they'd already embraced instead of going the other way around. There it was. To me calling those diets Word of Wisdom diets was like trying to fit the stepsister's foot into a glass slipper. It was a very nice glass slipper, but it was on the wrong foot and it would never really fit.

Over the years I looked at a number of diet programs and compared them to the Word of Wisdom. I looked at and occasionally considered the likes of low-fat diets, the grapefruit diet, the Pritikin program, the fat thermostat programs, the McDougal Diet, the Zone Diet, the Mediterranean Diet, The China Study, plant-based diets, paleo-diets, keto diets, and many more—looking for the perfect plan. There are numberless diet and so called healthy lifestyle plans to choose from. Most of the programs I looked at had good things to offer. But none was in its entirety quite right for me.

There was only one thing left to do: look at the Word of Wisdom itself and actually follow what it has to say. Then, I added one more component. I began to wonder if God had given us any other health advice in the scriptures. Is the Word of Wisdom the only and the last word on good health to which nothing should be added or taken away? Or can we find additional guidance as we study additional scriptures? After all, God has given guidance to his children from the beginning. How do the Bible and other scriptures support and augment what we have been given in the Doctrine and Covenants? So I began to search the scriptures, looking for insights.

But looking and seeing aren't always the same thing. We can be blinded by what we already believe and by what we think we know. If I had written a book on the Word of Wisdom thirty-five years ago, it would have been somewhat different from what I write today. In fact it too would have offered what is now a fairly PC diet, low in fat and high in complex carbs. I would have suggested limiting the amount of red meat in the diet, and may have suggested adding back butter and eggs. But over the years I have come to see things a little differently and, I hope, in a more complete way than I did then.

This book describes my thinking on the Word of Wisdom and its implementation as my understanding has grown and evolved over the last fifty years. It also touches on present scientific thinking in support of the Word of Wisdom. And it takes a look at what God has given us from the Bible and other scriptural sources beyond the Doctrine and Covenants as it relates to health and nutrition. He has not been silent!

1 BACKGROUND

What is the Word of Wisdom?

The Word of Wisdom is a gift from our Heavenly Father, given to us for both our physical and spiritual benefit. It is a health guide with spiritual promises. The revelation found in Section 89 of the Doctrine and Covenants was given by way of *greeting, not by commandment or constraint.* It is a loving suggestion showing the order and will of God, and like any suggestion it is left up to us to follow it or not. But, those who follow its suggestions will be healthier, stronger, and feel closer to the Spirit. Think about that!

The Word of Wisdom is not a moral law nor is it a plan of physical deprivation. It is a guide to good health. It was not given to restrict us in what we do, but to make our lives fuller, healthier and more abundant. It offers blessings of abundance both in the foods we eat and in the physical and spiritual health we can enjoy.

But even when we want to follow the plan the Lord has given us it is not always easy to understand what we should do; nor is it easy to make basic lifestyle changes. How can we implement long-term changes in how we think about food and in what we eat on a daily basis? How do we implement long-term changes in what our loved ones, our spouses and our children eat? (As every wife and mother knows, that's part of the battle—what those around us eat affects what and how we cook and eat.)

In this book I will break the Word of Wisdom down into steps that can be analyzed and then incorporated a little at a time over a period of weeks or months. The path to success lies in adopting this dietary plan over time, little by little, line upon line, and precept upon precept. When you reach the end you will have the tools you need to change your way of thinking, your way of eating and your lifestyle. I will briefly discuss the science behind the Word of Wisdom, and finally, I will provide some recipes that work for me, but I hope you will add recipes that work for you and your family as well. If you choose to, you can turn straight to *Implementation* and later go back and browse through the background and nutritional rationale at your leisure. I hope you will use this book in the way that works best for you.

Remember, the Word of Wisdom was not given as a commandment and for nearly a century it was most often seen as important advice but not as something required for temple worthiness. (2) Brigham Young declined to make the Word of Wisdom a test of fellowship or of membership in the church way back in 1861, explaining that, "Some of the brethren are very strenuous upon the Word of Wisdom and would like to have me preach upon it, and urge it upon the brethren, and make it a test of fellowship. I do not think I shall do so." (3) Even today only a part of the Word of Wisdom is mandated; living the whole Word of Wisdom is an individual choice and should remain so. It is something we can decide to follow or not. The blessings we choose to receive are up to us.

With the exodus to the Great Basin beginning in 1848, the Saints were plenty busy crossing the plains to Utah, taming the desert, and settling the surrounding territories. They had plenty to do, but abstaining from tobacco, alcohol, coffee and tea was not necessarily on their to-do-lists, and neither was temple attendance. The Word of Wisdom was not a part of a temple interview. Why? For one thing, there were no temples in operation in Utah or anywhere else on earth from the time the Saints left Nauvoo until the Saint George temple was dedicated thirty years later, in 1877. (Endowment houses filled the gap to some degree until temples were completed.) There was a lot going on, and the Church and its members had more to think about than temple recommends and the Word of Wisdom during those early years.

Still, Brigham Young, as President of the Church in September 1851, proposed in General Conference that all Saints formally covenant to abstain from tea, coffee, tobacco, whiskey and all things mentioned in the Word of Wisdom. That motion was accepted unanimously as a binding commandment for all church members. (4) The emphasis in following the Word of Wisdom at that time and up until the present day has been on abstaining from specific substances that are not good for the body as opposed to choosing the foods that are good and healthy for us. Abstaining from harmful substances has blessed the church and its members for generations. However the revelation addresses healthy as well as harmful substances—what we should eat and what we should avoid.

After 1851 the emphasis for members of the Church to abstain from coffee, tea, tobacco, and alcohol as mentioned in the Word of Wisdom grew at a fairly slow pace. By 1898 President Wilford Woodruff, commenting on the Word of Wisdom, noted that he regarded it in its entirety as given of the Lord for the Latter-day Saints to observe. But he cautioned bishops against withholding temple recommends from persons who did not adhere strictly to it. (5)

In an effort to help members live the Word of Wisdom, and as another step toward better implementation, the Council of the Twelve declared in 1905, that no man should hold a leadership position in the church if he would not obey the Word of Wisdom; and in 1906, the church officially introduced the use water in place of wine in the sacrament to better keep the spirit of the Word of

Wisdom. (6)

Joseph F. Smith believed that a long period of implementation was necessary in order to allow people "to overcome addictions to the noxious substances" named in the Word of Wisdom. He went on to explain, "the reason undoubtedly why the Word of Wisdom was given as not by 'commandment' or 'restraint' was that at that time at least, if it had been given as a commandment it would have brought every man and woman addicted to the use of these noxious things under condemnation; so the Lord was merciful and gave them a chance to overcome, before He brought them under the law." (7) President Smith recognized that the need to change practices deeply ingrained in cultural habits and in family traditions would take time.

So for several generations Latter-day Saint leaders taught the Word of Wisdom as a commandment but tolerated a variety of viewpoints on how strictly the commandment should be observed. Hot drinks were clarified as coffee and tea; the use of alcohol was first defined as spirits, and then expanded to all alcoholic beverages. As a church the Saints were given time to develop new traditions and our own culture of abstinence from habit-forming substances in order to sustain and make compliance easier. We see the culture and tradition of abstinence active in the church today. Adherence to the Word of Wisdom has made us unique as a church and stronger individually and as a people.

By 1919, with five temples in full operation and one soon to be opened in Mesa, Arizona, temple attendance had become a more regular feature of Latter-day Saint worship. In that year Heber J Grant called on all Saints to live the Word of Wisdom to the letter by abstaining from alcohol, coffee, tea, and tobacco, and included observation of the Word of Wisdom as defined in 1851 by President Young as part of the temple recommend interview. (8) We've done pretty well as a group in avoiding the negatives of the Word of Wisdom.

When will we as Saints be ready to take the next step in fully living the Word of Wisdom and experience the increased blessings it promises us? And what does the next step entail? To find out what the Word of Wisdom has to say concerning nutrition and diet we need to read the Word of Wisdom, perhaps with new eyes, and we need to learn how to adopt what it offers us. A period of implementation may be necessary, just as it was with the "do not's" of the Word of Wisdom, as we make changes to our personal and family cultures, traditions and diet choices, and move forward. However, for those committed to eating the Lord's way a period of weeks or months should be sufficient to develop a practical, healthy, productive lifestyle and diet plan in accordance with the guidelines and suggestions the Lord has given us.

The greater part of the Word of Wisdom is a guide to healthy eating which, when followed (along with the admonition to avoid certain harmful substances), promises us individually a healthy life. Indeed those who remember to keep and do these sayings are promised health, strength, wisdom and great treasures of knowledge—even hidden treasures. We are promised that we shall run and not be weary, and walk and not faint, but only if we are actually running and walking. Finally we are promised that the destroying angel shall pass us by and not slay us. We will not be cut down before our time.

Remember, God wants us to care for and nourish both our body and our spirit. After all, our body is home to our spirit and for that reason alone needs to be kept in good repair. I listened to a six-year-old bear her testimony not too long ago. She explained in her sweet voice, "Every morning while I'm eating breakfast my mom reads the Book of Mormon to me from her phone so that when I go to school I'll have a little piece of the spirit in my heart." And I thought, What a wise mother to provide double nourishment every morning at breakfast. Let's not neglect either the body or the spirit, but keep a "little piece of the spirit" in our hearts every day!

2 DOCTRINE & COVENANTS, SECTION 89

Revelation given through Joseph Smith the Prophet, at Kirtland, Ohio, February 27, 1833. As a consequence of the early brethren using tobacco in their meetings, the Prophet was led to ponder upon the matter; consequently, he inquired of the Lord concerning it. This revelation, known as the Word of Wisdom, was the result:

The use of wine, strong drinks, tobacco, and hot drinks is proscribed; Herbs, fruits, flesh, and grain are ordained for the use of man and of animals; Obedience to gospel law, including the Word of Wisdom, brings temporal and spiritual blessings.

1 A Word of Wisdom, for the benefit of the council of high priests, assembled in Kirtland, and the church, and also the saints in Zion—

2 To be sent greeting; not by commandment or constraint, but by revelation and the word of wisdom, showing forth the order and will of God in the temporal salvation of all saints in the last days—

3 Given for a principle with promise, adapted to the capacity of the weak and the weakest of all saints, who are or can be called saints.

4 Behold, verily, thus saith the Lord unto you: In consequence of evils and designs which do and will exist in the hearts of conspiring men in the last days, I have warned you, and forewarn you, by giving unto you this word of wisdom by revelation—

5 That inasmuch as any man drinketh wine or strong drink among you, behold it is not good, neither meet in the sight of your Father, only in assembling yourselves together to offer up your sacraments before him.

6 And, behold, this should be wine, yea, pure wine of the grape of the vine, of your own make.

7 And, again, strong drinks are not for the belly, but for the washing of your bodies.

8 And again, tobacco is not for the body, neither for the belly, and is not good for man, but is an herb for bruises and all sick cattle, to be used with judgment and skill.

9 And again, hot drinks are not for the body or belly.

10 And again, verily I say unto you, all wholesome herbs God hath ordained for the constitution, nature, and use of man—

11 Every herb in the season thereof, and every fruit in the season thereof; all these to be used with prudence and thanksgiving.

12 Yea, flesh also of beasts and of the fowls of the air, I, the Lord, have ordained for the use of man with thanksgiving; nevertheless they are to be used sparingly;

13 And it is pleasing unto me that they should not be used, only in times of winter, or of cold, or famine.

14 All grain is ordained for the use of man and of beasts, to be the staff of life, not only for man but for the beasts of the field, and the fowls of heaven, and all wild animals that run or creep on the earth;

15 And these hath God made for the use of man only in times of famine and excess of hunger.

16 All grain is good for the food of man; as also the fruit of the vine; that which yieldeth fruit, whether in the ground or above the ground—

17 Nevertheless, wheat for man, and corn for the ox, and oats for the horse, and rye for the fowls and for swine, and for all beasts of the field, and barley for all useful animals, and for mild drinks, as also other grain.

18 And all saints who remember to keep and do these sayings, walking in obedience to the commandments, shall receive health in their navel and marrow to their bones;

19 And shall find wisdom and great treasures of knowledge, even hidden treasures;

20 And shall run and not be weary, and shall walk and not faint.

21 And I, the Lord, give unto them a promise, that the destroying angel shall pass by them, as the children of Israel, and not slay them. Amen.

The Word of Wisdom is only twenty-one verses in total. The first nine verses deal with what not to eat or ingest. We'll start with verse ten, 'all wholesome herbs God hath ordained for the constitution, nature, and use of man—'

3 NUTRITIONAL DEFINITIONS

We're almost ready to begin our study and analysis of the Word of Wisdom, but before we get started let's review some basic nutritional terms. Many nutritionists classify food into three basic nutrient groups: Protein, fats and carbohydrates. I am listing two additional essential nutrients that I think, after you've read through what I have to say, you'll agree with: Protein, fats, carbohydrates, *fiber* and *water*. Understanding what these nutrients are, how they affect our bodies and our health, and why each one is essential to our well-being is important in understanding the importance of the Word of Wisdom. So let's define each one quickly.

Protein: The word protein comes from a Greek word meaning *of first importance*. Protein is made up of complex chains of amino acids. Amino acids, the building blocks of protein, are not only important; they are essential to almost every chemical reaction in the human body. Protein is essential for the building of skin, bones, and muscles as well as less obvious but equally important components of our bodies including hormones and neurotransmitters. The DNA in our chromosomes is built of specific proteins. Protein makes us who we are.

Not all proteins are the same for humans. Proteins from animal sources (with the exceptions of seafood and the whey and casein from milk) are more likely to encourage the growth of pathogenic bacteria in the gut, adversely affecting overall health. Fish, eggs, cheese, nuts and legumes are all good sources of protein. Plant proteins in particular seem to encourage beneficial intestinal bacteria.

When protein is broken down into individual amino acids during digestion the body is able to reassemble those amino acids in various ways. However, there are nine amino acids out of the twenty-one our body uses that cannot be reconstructed from existing materials; those amino acids are called *essential*. We have to get them from what we eat. The body can't fabricate these essential amino acids so it is important to eat foods that contain them.

We need protein every day in every meal, and our need for protein actually increases as we get older. Eat more, not less protein! But don't eat too much at any one time. The body can only absorb a little protein at a time, so eat some protein with every meal. Protein triggers only a slight release of insulin as it is digested, so it can help in the control of body weight and diabetes.

Fat: The fats and oils we eat are broken down into glycerol and fatty acids. As with proteins, there are *essential* fatty acids, or in other words, fatty acids that the body cannot synthesize by recombining other fatty acids. We are dependent on diet to provide our brain and body with the essential fatty acids the body can't produce by itself. We need fat and it is important to eat fats that provide the essential fatty acids we require.

Why is fat important? Our brains are made up of 60% fat, and unless we have enough healthy fats in our diet the brain cannot function efficiently. Cutting back on dietary fat affects the overall health of both the brain and body—our mental and physical well-being.

Fat is found in meat, fish, eggs, dairy products, seeds and nuts. The oils pressed from olives and other seeds and nuts, including coconuts and grape seeds, are one hundred percent healthy fat. Heat processed oils, on the other hand, are lacking in nutrients and can put the body out of balance. Most relatively clear vegetable oils, i.e. corn oil, canola oil and the many other vegetable oil available are heat processed. I will talk more about oils later. But remember, healthy pressed oils are a necessary part of a healthy diet.

Another benefit from fat: Fats do **not** trigger the release of insulin and so they help keep blood sugar in balance. As paradoxical as it may seem, low fat diets contribute to obesity while higher fat diets can contribute to weight loss, but only when the essential nutrients are in the proper balance. Animal fats such as cream, butter, lard, tallow, etc. should be avoided, while vegetable fats such as olive oil, coconut oil, avocado oils and some others, are all good sources of dietary fat. We need some fat every day with every meal.

Carbohydrates: Carbohydrates include sugars and starches. Starches are made up of long chains of sugar molecules and are sometimes called complex carbohydrates. Caloric sweeteners or sugars, and refined white flour are simple carbohydrates. Fruits, vegetables, legumes and grains are all sources of complex carbohydrates, but there are differences in what each of these provides the body. Vegetables tend to have a low carbohydrate load but are rich in vitamins, minerals, water and fiber. Fruits are generally a denser source of carbohydrates than vegetables but provide a fairly sizeable amount of water and fiber along with fructose or fruit sugar. Legumes—beans and peas—carry a high load of fiber and a moderate amount of protein as well as carbohydrates. Whole grains have a moderate carbohydrate load and are rich in vitamins, minerals, some oil, and fiber.

When people talk about avoiding carbs they are usually referring to simple carbohydrates, refined sugars and enriched white flour. Both sugar and white flour are refined from vegetable sources or whole grains, but the beneficial nutrients, oils and fiber have been removed. All simple carbohydrates trigger insulin and raise blood sugar. The oils and fiber that would normally buffer the insulin load and enhance digestion have been removed. Refined caloric sweeteners, including all forms of sugar no matter the color, as well as corn syrup, high fructose corn syrup, agave syrup, and others, provide sucrose or fructose, which breaks down rapidly into glucose. Glucose from these sources quickly enters the blood stream, carrying with it no beneficial nutrients and none of the buffering affect of fiber. White flour is also quickly converted into glucose and enters the blood stream along with a dozen or so enriching synthetic vitamins, but without fiber or oil's buffer found in whole grain.

Fiber: Fiber consists of non-digestible plant material. While often classified as a carbohydrate, fiber passes through the body without an immediate impact on blood sugar and without adding calories. We cannot digest fiber directly, but the bacteria in our intestines use fiber and its byproducts to make the vitamins, enzymes and other compounds that are essential to the proper digestion of our food.

Fiber is only found in plants. There is no fiber in animal food sources. Fiber is classified as soluble and non-soluble. Both are necessary for the good health of the gut and our friendly little gut bacteria. Because the body cannot produce fiber it is an essential nutrient, necessary for proper digestion and good health. We have to eat it to enjoy its positive effects, and it is only found in plants.

Water: Water is defined as an essential nutrient because we require it in greater amounts than the body can produce. All biochemical reactions in the body occur in water. Water fills the spaces between cells and helps form the large molecules we need including proteins and glycogen. We need water everyday. Don't count on sugary or artificially sweetened drinks to provide your body with the water it needs long term. It often takes additional water to fully metabolize both sugary and artificially sweetened drinks.

And finally, just a note on **insulin**. Insulin, a hormone produced in the pancreas, regulates the amount of glucose in the blood. Insulin is what allows your body to use glucose for energy or to store glucose as fat for future energy. The best way to gain weight is to eat foods that trigger insulin. And the opposite is also true. The best way to lose weight is to eat foods that don't trigger insulin—it is impossible to gain weight or store fat without insulin.

Carbohydrates, especially simple carbohydrates, trigger insulin; protein causes a slight release of insulin. Fats do not trigger insulin at all. Paradoxical as it may seem, a diet made up only of fats would cause rapid weight loss. But it probably wouldn't be healthy and is not recommended!

Type II diabetes is caused by an insulin imbalance. When the body loses its sensitivity to insulin it can't process glucose correctly and blood glucose levels become and remain elevated, causing the release of more ineffective insulin. The excess glucose in the blood, rather than meeting the body's energy needs, gets processed and stored as fat. It's a vicious cycle, leaving a body feeling weaker, hungrier and heavier.

Obesity is often cited as the cause of type II diabetes, but in fact both obesity and diabetes are symptoms of insulin imbalance; insulin imbalance is the cause of both. Confusing a symptom with the cause makes no sense. Both need to be correctly understood and treated. (9)

Remember, all carbohydrates trigger the release of insulin, and simple carbohydrates especially raise blood sugar; protein triggers insulin slightly; fat and fiber do not trigger insulin at all.. The cream in ice cream as an example, buffers the sugar in ice cream giving it an overall lower glycemic index number than cakes or cookies, which consist mostly of refined flour and sugars. If you must choose one, eat the ice cream and leave the cake behind! Better yet, look to the Word of Wisdom and find a healthier way to live.

In reality it is best to avoid simple carbs even in combination with healthier nutrients. Fiber, fat, protein, and complex carbohydrates buffer the absorption and slow the release of glucose (and thus insulin) into the bloodstream. Insulin stimulates the cells of the body to absorb glucose from the blood stream, but when insulin is out of balance or when too much glucose is dumped into the blood stream all at once, it wreaks havoc with blood sugar levels. Complex carbohydrates are naturally buffered with fiber, water, oil, and even protein in every bite.

We need all five of the essential nutrients everyday in combination with each other. We can't live on water or oil alone, nor can we live on protein, fiber or carbohydrates alone. These nutrients work together and each one should a part of our daily diet, preferably at every meal.

Now let's jump into the Word of Wisdom itself.

4 HERBS AND FRUITS

*10 And again, verily I say unto you, **all wholesome herbs** God hath ordained for the constitution, nature, and use of man— **11 Every herb in the season thereof, and every fruit in the season thereof**; all these to be used with prudence and thanksgiving.*

Verses 10 and 11 name two food groups: wholesome herbs and fruits. What exactly are herbs? The Oxford English Dictionary defines herb as: *a plant of which the stem does not become woody and persistent but remains more or less soft and succulent.* In other words, all those edible leafy green plants that don't grow into trees.

In the 1800s the word *herb* was used to mean any green plant (excluding trees) comprehending vegetables and all green herbage. So wholesome herbs are edible plants we more commonly refer to as vegetables, or what we think of as leafy green vegetables today. The Word of Wisdom starts off right here recommending that we eat leafy green vegetables in season and fruit. These should make up the foundation of our diet.

Do the scriptures say anything else about fruits and vegetables? In Genesis in the Bible, in the beginning we're given the very same counsel we have in the Doctrine and Covenants:

And God said, Behold, I have given you every herb bearing seed, which is upon the face of all the earth, and every tree in the which is the fruit of a tree yielding seed; to you it shall be for meat. And to every beast of the earth, and to every fowl of the air, and to everything that creepeth upon the earth, wherein there is life I have given every green herb for meat: and it was so. (Genesis 1: 29, 30)

(Note that *meat* in these verses means food in general, not animal flesh. This is a common use of the word *meat* in the scriptures and especially in the Bible.) Adam and Eve were given the same dietary advice we received through the Prophet Joseph Smith: eat fruits and leafy green vegetables.

Did you think for a minute that Genesis 1:30 was going to say that every beast and fowl was also given to us for meat? Nope. It doesn't go there. Humans are omnivores. We can eat plants and we can eat meat. But we are mostly designed for a plant-based and soft food menu. Just look in your mouth—we have twenty molars, eight incisors and four canines. The molars are grinding teeth for chewing herbs, fruits, legumes and grains. The incisors are biting teeth for biting into relatively soft foods like apples or celery or eggs; and the four canines are tearing teeth for meat and stubborn packaging.

We are not carnivores. Carnivores have mostly tearing teeth; the carnivore's jaws move vertically, up and down to facilitate ripping and tearing. Our jaw moves both vertically and horizontally to crush and chew. Twenty-eight of our thirty-two teeth are designed to accommodate a plant diet. In addition humans have the relatively long intestinal tract designed for plant digestion. Our stomachs are less acidic than a carnivores' stomach, and our saliva is alkaline to assist in the breakdown of carbohydrates and plant nutrients. Our bodies are not designed for a diet made up primarily of meat and meat fats. In fact it takes large amounts of uric acid for our digestive system to break animal protein down into useable amino acids. Large amounts of uric acid are toxic to our bodies and accelerate aging. Nobody likes that!

No wonder the Designer started off by telling us to eat leafy green vegetables and fruit. Biologically meat should not be a major part of our diet. Leafy green vegetables and fruits are both high in fiber content and nutrients, but fairly low in simple carbohydrates. They're just what we need.

In Deuteronomy, the Lord described the Promised Land to the Israelites who had wandered in the wilderness for forty years:

> *Therefore thou shalt keep the commandments of the LORD thy God to walk in his ways, and to fear him. For the LORD thy God bringeth thee into a good land, a land of brooks of water, of fountains and depths that spring out of valleys and hills; A land of wheat and barley, and vines, and fig trees, and pomegranates; a land of olive oil, and honey. (Deuteronomy 8: 8, 9)*

What did the Israelites look forward to coming out of the desert? A land of fresh water, grains, fruit, vines, olive oil and honey, and undoubtedly leafy greens, a lovely land. As the Israelites approached the land of Canaan, their promised land, Moses sent men ahead to explore and,

> *When they reached the Valley of Eshkol, they cut off a branch bearing a single cluster of grapes. Two of them carried it on a pole between them, along with some pomegranates and figs. (Numbers 13: 23)*

That must have been some grape cluster to require two men and a pole to carry it. This was one of the signs that they'd reached the end of their time in the desert. They were coming to a pleasant land. Apples, apricots, berries, melons, dates and raisins are just a few of the fruits they may have encountered as mentioned in the Bible. Citrus fruits and pineapple were common in the Middle East and were undoubtedly abundant in the Promised Land as well. And just in case you wondered, it may not say *leafy greens* anywhere in the Bible, but it does talk about bitter herbs, which included many of the vegetables we would classify as leafy greens today—lettuce, chicory, mustard, radishes, mandrake, peppermint, snakeroot, and dandelion to name a few. Certainly enough greens to make a decent salad! Today we are fortunate to have access to fresh fruits and vegetables including leafy greens from around the world. We live in an abundant, even a bountiful time.

Again in the Bible we read about Abigail, a woman who lived at the time of King David:

> *Then Abigail made haste, and took two hundred loaves, and two bottles of wine, and five sheep ready dressed, and five measures of parched corn, and an hundred clusters of raisins, and two hundred cakes of figs, and laid them on asses. (I Samuel 25: 18)*

Abigail was trying to appease King David with her gifts in a time of war. What better way than with food? She brought not only fresh fruit but also dried raisins and corn (grain), and fruit cooked into fig cakes. And a fruit drink!

We read about fruit and raisins again when David was traveling:

> *And when David was a little past the top of the hill,*

behold, Ziba, the servant of Mephibosheth, met him with a couple of asses saddled and upon them two hundred loaves of bread, a hundred bunches raisins, and a hundred of summer fruits, and a bottle of wine. And the king said unto Ziba, What meanest thou by these? And Ziba said, The asses be for the king's household to ride on; and the bread and summer fruit for the young men to eat; and the wine, that such as be faint in the wilderness may drink.   (2 Samuel 16:1, 2)

When King David was on the move, when fresh fruit may have been difficult to transport, he was given raisin cakes and fig cakes. But later he was given summer fruits. In both instances the men received a fairly small amount of wine, one or two bottles, and soldiers were able to get along with bread and fruit.

When David and his men were pursuing a raiding party they came upon a hungry man without food or drink:

They found an Egyptian in the field and brought him to David, and gave him bread, and he did eat; and they made him drink— And they gave him a piece of a cake of figs and two clusters of raisins: and when he had eaten, his spirit came again to him: for he had eaten no bread, nor drunk any water, three days and three nights. (1 Samuel 30: 11-12)

Water and fruitcakes. I imagine the cakes may have been

something like our fig newton's or banana, pumpkin and nut breads if we made them with whole wheat flour and a little honey, but not quite as soft or sweet, not nearly as refined as what we might call cakes today.

Reread this description of the Promised Land:

> *For the Lord thy God bringeth thee into a good land, a land of brooks of water, of fountains and depths that spring out of valleys and hills; A land of wheat and barley and vines and fig trees and pomegranates; a land of olive and honey; A land wherein thou shalt eat bread without scarceness, thou shalt not lack any thing in it; a land whose stones are iron, and out of whose hills thou mayest dig brass. When thou hast eaten and art full, then thou shalt bless the Lord thy God for the good land which he hath given thee. (Deuteronomy 8: 7-10)*

It sounds so good. Of course the verses in Deuteronomy 8 mention several nutritious foods besides leafy greens and fruit. But let's not get ahead of ourselves. There are many references to fruits and vegetables in the Bible. And from the Word of Wisdom we know that leafy green vegetables and fruits are not only pleasing and delicious, they are the foundation of the Lord's diet plan, something we can eat every day.

EAT LEAFY GREEN VEGETABLES AND FRUITS

5 THE FLESH OF BEASTS AND FOWLS

12 *Yea, **flesh also of beasts and of the fowls of the air**, I, the Lord, have ordained for the use of man with thanksgiving; nevertheless **they are to be used sparingly**;*

13And it is pleasing unto me that they should not be used, only in times of winter, or of cold, or famine.

14 *All grain is ordained for the use of man and of beasts, to be the staff of life, not only for man but for **the beasts of the field, and the fowls of heaven, and all wild animals that run or creep on the earth;***

15 And these hath God made for the use of man only in times of famine and excess of hunger.

The Word of Wisdom is very clear that the flesh of beasts and fowls, and in fact of ALL wild animals that run or creep on the earth, is to be used sparingly. And it is pleasing to the Lord that they should NOT be used at all except in times of winter, or of cold or of famine. Verse 15 reemphasizes what must be an important point: *And these (beasts and fowls) God has made for our use ONLY in times of famine or excess hunger.* This doesn't just say eat red meat sparingly. It says **don't eat red meat or chicken or turkey, or the flesh of any other animal that runs upon the earth, unless you don't have anything else to eat.**

Joseph Fielding Smith commented on our position with regard to eating meat: "While it is ordained that the flesh of animals is for man's food, yet this should be used sparingly. The wording of this revelation is perfectly clear in relation to this subject, but we do not always heed it". (10)

But didn't the people in Biblical times eat meat? They did. Soldiers in the field ate meat if it was available. When the prodigal son returned home his father hurried to cook a fatted calf. Beef was eaten in times of war and celebration—weddings, homecomings, and other festive occasions. Lamb was prepared and eaten at Passover.

But during Biblical times animals were not raised strictly for meat, nor was meat eaten regularly. Sheep and goats were raised for both the wool and milk they provided, while cattle or oxen were raised as beasts of burden, as a source of leather, and for milk. And animals were also kept for sacrificial purposes, looking forward to the great sacrifice of Jesus Christ who was to come.

Jesus Christ undoubtedly followed Levitical law and would have eaten a diet rich in whole grains, fruits, vegetables and fish. He would have also eaten ritually clean or kosher meat and poultry, but these would not have been a major part of his diet. Christ's main source of animal protein was fish.

So what about fish? Do fish run or creep on the earth? I don't think so. But you can decide for yourself whether you think fish are included in verses 12 through 15. Nevertheless, the Bible and the Law of Moses are clear when it came to eating fish:

> *These shall ye eat of all that are in the waters: whatsoever hath fins and scales in the waters, in the seas, and in the rivers, them shall ye eat. And all that have not fins and scales in the seas, and in the rivers, of all that move in the waters, and of any living thing which is in the water; they shall be an abomination unto you. Whatsoever hath no fins nor scales in the waters that shall be an abomination unto you. (Leviticus 11: 9-12)*

The Bible mentions fish over and over again. If it has fins and scales, it's good to eat. Why doesn't the Word of Wisdom mention fish? Could it be because the Lord has already told us in the Bible that fish is a healthy, nutritious food and He didn't see a need to repeat himself in this modern revelation? Could it be that in the mid 1800s fish was such a common, everyday food choice that no one would have grouped fish with creatures that run, fly or crawl?

During Christ's lifetime people in the land of Israel would have eaten a wide variety of fish from the Sea of Galilee, from the Mediterranean, from the River Jordan, and from other rivers and bodies of water. But they would not have eaten shellfish or sharks, or dolphins or whales. Those animals were ritually unclean. (When I refer to the Law of Moses's dietary laws from here on or when I use the term kosher to refer to "clean" or acceptable foods, I am not suggesting that we return to the rituals attached to the kosher laws in the Old Testament. But I do believe that as dietary guidelines the kosher laws are still generally valid.)

As a follower of the Law of Moses, Jesus would have eaten meat only from cud chewing animals with a cloven hoof. These could have included cattle, sheep, goats and deer. He would not have eaten pork at any time, nor would he have eaten visible fat on any meat. Fat was carefully trimmed away when meat was prepared for cooking, and rendered fats like lard were not considered clean and were not used as a food or in foods. (Rendered fats could be used acceptably in things like skin salves, medicines, and lamp oil.) The skin of chickens and other fowls was also removed before the meat was cooked. Blood was unclean, not to be eaten at any time. Leviticus 7: 23-24 is very clear:

> *Speak unto the children of Israel saying, Ye shall eat no manner of fat, of ox, or of sheep, or of goat. And the fat of the beast that dieth of itself, and the fat of that which is torn with beasts, may be used in any other use; but ye shall in no wise eat it.*

Don't eat the fat! Don't eat the fat from slaughtered animals or from dead or damaged animals. Don't eat any of it. You can use it to treat dry skin, or to make soaps, or for any external purpose, but don't eat it. Proverbs 23 calls rich and fatty foods deceitful foods:

> When thou sittest to eat with a ruler, consider diligently what is before thee; Be not desirous of his dainties; for they are deceitful meat. Hear thou my son and be wise, and guide thine heart in the way. Be not among winebibbers; among riotous eaters of flesh. (Proverbs 23: 1,3, 19-20)

So if meat was only eaten sparingly and only after careful preparation what else did the people of the Bible eat? Loaves and fishes were such a common meal in Biblical times that it comes as no surprise that Jesus refers to loaves and fishes various times in the New Testament.

Lehi and his descendants in the Book of Mormon also followed the Law of Moses both in animal sacrifice and the dietary guidelines. In I Nephi 2 at the very beginning of the Book of Mormon Lehi offers sacrifice. In chapter 4, Nephi, as he stands over Laban, tells us:

> Yea, and I also thought that they (his posterity) could not keep the commandments of the Lord according to the law of Moses, save they should have the law.

He is not simply concerned with the Ten Commandments.

The dietary and sacrificial laws were specific and complex. They needed the Books of Moses to comply fully with those laws. They kept the sacrificial laws up until the time the Savior appeared to them in the New World after Christ's resurrection. In Jarom 1: 5, 6 the condition of the people is described:

> *Two hundred years had passed away, and the people of Nephi . . . observed to keep the law of Moses. . . and the Lamanites. . . loved murder and would drink the blood of beasts.*

Drinking the blood of beasts? Definitely against the dietary laws. Again in II Nephi 5: 24, the Lamanites are described as:

> " . . . an idle people, full of mischief and subtlety, and did seek in the wilderness for beasts of prey."

Along with all the other problems the Nephites ascribed to the Lamanites, they were hunting and eating ritually unclean animals. This description makes me think of an imagined neighbor, a lazy troublemaker, who sits on his porch in his underwear AND drinks beer. We don't drink beer. So drinking beer is one more strike against that lazy fellow who is neither living the Word of Wisdom nor working as hard as we are. And he is already hard to get along with. For the Nephites the fact that the Lamanites ate beasts of prey was one more proof that they did not keep the commandments and could not be considered good neighbors.

Obviously, considering what the Word of Wisdom has to say, we need to be careful about what types of meat we choose to eat. I avoid meat; instead I've added fish to my meals. I used to think I didn't like fish much, but I've begun to enjoy it. (I still think of my Thanksgiving turkey as that fatted calf which is only prepared rarely and on very special occasions. While I try not to find too many special occasions throughout the year, there are a few worth celebrating!)

As He was in former days, the Lord is merciful with us today. He has not created a hard and fast standard for meat consumption. Each of us individually, with our own conscience must settle the matter for ourselves as to what constitutes *sparingly,* or *only in times of famine or excess hunger.*

"But," you may say, "*Bacon (*substitute any other cut of meat here*) tastes so good.*" And it does, and that's also what folks say who want a glass of wine with their dinner. It may taste good; it may be what they're used to eating; it may even be what their mother and grannie always served, but that doesn't change the wording of the Word of Wisdom.

So what is the problem with meat? Meat gets both good and bad health reviews: meat is an excellent source of vitamins, minerals and nutrients we need for good health. For more than fifty years meat, along with saturated fat, was demonized as the cause of heart disease. But in the past few years over seventy reputable, published studies dispute those now outdated findings. In fact, when saturated fats are replaced with an increased consumption of simple carbohydrates, there is an increased risk of coronary heart disease and overall mortality from all causes. (11) In addition, with increased simple carbohydrate consumption there is an increased incidence of inflammation and a trend to impaired glucose tolerance, higher body fat, weight gain and an increase in rates of diabetes. Something is wrong with the typical American diet but it's more complicated than the amount of meat or saturated fat we eat.

In some studies both red meat and poultry have been linked to an increased risk of cancer. But let me say here that the data from food studies and food trials are remarkably unreliable for a number of reasons. Food intake in most food trials is self-reported: This group of people say they eat very little meat, or no fat or reduced sugar. But there is nobody coming into the kitchen to verify what is eaten, how often, or how it's prepared.

In addition, it is almost impossible to alter one component of the diet without changing other aspects of the diet. I may cut red meat out of my diet, but I will substitute for the loss of that food by eating a greater amount of something else. Are the observed health consequences a result of eliminating meat or because of the increased consumption of vegetables or beans or whatever other inevitable changes were made to compensate for my removing meat?

And finally food studies in the past fifty years were often carried out or paid for by biased entities like Coca Cola or Proctor and Gamble who had a vested interest in the results. This was most blatantly seen with tobacco studies in the last century. But it undoubtedly continues today.

John P.A. Ioannidis, a respected faculty member at Stanford University, published a paper in 2005 titled *Why Most Published Research Findings are False*. (12) It sounds like it should be a joke, but unfortunately it's no joking matter. In 2012 Ioannidis coauthored a paper showing that pretty much everything in the refrigerator has been shown to both cause and prevent cancer. (13) That's the way food studies work.

We need a better guide. And fortunately we do have a better guide. Nutritional studies may or may not support the elimination of meat from the diet. A similar case can and has been made for and against coffee. You can look up studies that show whatever you hope to find. The scientific research is unclear as to whether coffee drinking is healthy or unhealthy. Nevertheless we trust the Word of Wisdom and the covenants we've made and we choose not to drink coffee. We can make the same decision for meat.

It has been reported that pescetarians (vegetarians who also eat fish) who eat fish at least once a month, have lower cancer rates and overall greater cancer protection than meat eaters. In another study eating fish as the only source of animal protein reportedly cut the risk of certain types of cancer by 50%—by half (14). That is a huge percentage. (But, could the results also be attributed to the vegetarian/non-processed food diet? Food trials are tricky.) Remember, you can find studies that support almost any position. Darn it!

Finally, another long-term study conducted in Finland found that consumption of all animal protein increased the risk of cancers except for consumption of fish and eggs. Fish and eggs were both found to be beneficial! (15) I liked what these studies said so I included them!

Recent studies have shown that red meat increases the numbers of inflammatory bacteria species in the gut, and that the protein from animal sources (except milk proteins) encourages the growth of pathogenic bacteria. When you eat a lot of meat and animal fat you are feeding inflammatory, bile tolerant microbes.

Interestingly the milk proteins casein and whey have the opposite effects, reducing intestinal inflammation and increasing the production of anti-inflammatory short chain fatty acids. Yea Milk!!But saturated fats, including milk fats, tend to have a negative effect on the microbiome. So drink milk, but skip the fat!

Monounsaturated fats like those in fatty fish and many plant foods have a neutral or beneficial effect. These studies conclude that vegetable and seafood fats are healthier for us, better for the microbiome, and lower our levels of inflammation—the opposite of what saturated animal fat does. Imagine that! Maybe we can trust God!

Regardless, I've wondered whether it was for more than nutritional and digestive reasons that we are counseled not to eat meat. (Remember our long intestinal tract.) As I've pondered this I've begun to consider things that have little or nothing to do with nutrition.

In the Old Testament sheep, goats, cattle, doves and other animals were killed as a part of a religious rite. Animal sacrifice was performed with Christ's ultimate sacrifice in mind. The killing of animals was not something to be taken lightly. Death and the shedding of blood, even animal blood, were not taken lightly. The regulations for taking an animal's life were set out in the Bible along with the specific processes for sacrifice. Yet today we slaughter animals thoughtlessly. We rarely see the animal whose meat we consume. We rarely see the inhumane conditions many animals endure before being slung onto the meat hook. We almost never take the time to consider the sacrifice inherent in the meat we prepare or the greater sacrifice of Jesus Christ in this context. Perhaps killing and eating animal flesh is not the preferred way when other less cruel, less invasive means are available for us, means that incorporate better health and nutrition. Is this why we are asked not to eat meat except in times of cold or famine?

Isaiah 11: 7 indicates that during the millennium not even

carnivorous beasts will eat meat. "And the lion shall eat straw like the ox." Will we do any less?

Another factor to be considered is the levels of antibiotics and hormones currently used in commercially raised meat, both from beast and fowl. Certainly these additives have at best, untested and unhealthy effects. Is this why we're asked not to eat meat except in times of cold or famine? Animal sacrifice and antibiotics may have nothing to do with it. I do know that the Lord has counseled that it is better if we don't eat meat at all.

Maybe we should substitute fish as a good and healthy source of animal protein.

MEAT SHOULD BE EATEN SPARINGLY OR NOT AT ALL.

EAT FISH AS A HEALTHY ALTERNATIVE.

6 GRAINS, VINES AND ROOTS

14 All grain *is ordained for the use of man and of beasts, to be the staff of life, not only for man but for the beasts of the field, and the fowls of heaven, and all wild animals that run or creep on the earth;*

15 *And these hath God made for the use of man only in times of famine and excess of hunger.*

16 *All grain is good for the food of man; as also **the fruit of the vine; that which yieldeth fruit, whether in the ground or above the ground—***

17 *Nevertheless**, wheat for man**, and corn for the ox, and oats for the horse, and rye for the fowls and for swine, and for all beasts of the field, and barley for all useful animals, and for mild drinks, as also other grain.*

All grain is good for humans as food but **wheat** is specifically indicated as the grain for men and women. Wheat is of course whole wheat. That is the only way it will grow. I will say more about whole wheat later. Wheat and its byproduct gluten have gotten a bad rap recently, but wheat is the most cultivated and consumed plant in the entire world. Wheat supports human life around the globe and whole wheat bread is truly the staff of life. Bread is so common and so important to life that Christ compares himself to bread, telling us, *"I am the bread of life."* It is He who sustains us spiritually in the same way bread sustains us physically.

Grains that were common during the time of Christ include wheat, barley, millet, oats and rye, and all are still common today. We have access now to other grains that were unknown at the time of Christ, specifically maize corn and rice, but also other grain-like seeds like quinoa. We have ample choices when it comes to grain.

Luke 6: 1 refers to wheat:

> *And on the second Sabbath after the first, he went through the cornfields and his disciples plucked the ears of corn and did eat, rubbing them in their hands.*

Wait, that doesn't say wheat, it says corn. But remember, what we call corn today is the New World plant maize. Our corn or maize was nonexistent in the Old World at the time of Christ. The word *corn* as used in the Bible is a generic word for grain of all types. Because the disciples were hungry they went through a field of wheat and ate the raw grain. The same is true for the corn in the story of Joseph in Egypt with the seven ears of corn. Despite all those cute children's coloring books, it was wheat or some other Old World grain that Joseph saw in a dream and later grew and stored for the coming years of famine.

Wheat is mentioned by name at least fifty-one times in the Bible. In Genesis 30 the wheat harvest is mentioned. The barley harvest is mentioned in Ruth 1; but wheat was and is the king of grains, and as such was valued at three times the price of barley. (See Revelations 6:6) Bread, including wheat breads and breads made with other grains, is still one of the most common, important and ancient staple foods in the world.

So far the Word of Wisdom advises us to eat leafy green vegetables, fruit, fish instead of meat, and grain. Verse 16 adds the fruit of the vine. The **fruit of the vine** whether in the ground or above the ground is also good for food. What grows on vines? Above the ground: legumes—that is beans, peas, chickpeas, lentils, and so on—grapes, squash, melons and cucumbers, just to name a few plants. You can continue the list. Below the ground we have potatoes, yams, peanuts and many more vine growing vegetables.

In the Old Testament the Israelites, worried about leaving the security of Egypt, harkened back to the foods they enjoyed there:

> *We remember the fish, which we did eat in Egypt freely; the cucumbers, and the melons, and the leeks, and the onions, and the garlick (Numbers 11:5)*

Of course they were worried about leaving behind all those good fruits of the vine whether in the ground or above the ground. Of course they worried about leaving behind the fish. They were leaving the Nile River and going out into the desert where they would be on a fairly restricted diet. Garlic, onions, and leeks were so common in Egypt that they are depicted in pictographs on the walls of Egyptian tombs dating back more than 5000 years. It wasn't just Moses and the Children of Israel who looked on these foods with fondness!

And what about legumes or beans? They are certainly fruits of the vine. Remember Daniel? He chose to follow Levitical law rather than eat the rich meats and wine offered by the king. But what did Daniel eat instead? According to the Bible Daniel and his friends ate pulse and drank water. (Daniel 1:12)

Pulse? Pulse is pretty much the same food group as legumes. Pulse includes beans, peas, chickpeas, and lentils.

Whatever Daniel ate specifically, it consisted of wholesome herbs and a specific selection of fruits of the vine. And at the end of only ten days of sticking to this clean, kosher diet Daniel and his four friends were found to be *"ten times better than all the magicians and astrologers of the king"*. Better at what? Strength? Reasoning ability? Running speed? Vitality? It doesn't say, but he was ten times better at whatever it was—maybe all those things—after less than two weeks of healthy eating.

Daniel was not the only one who ate a diet of pulse. Everybody outside the court ate beans! When Esau sold his birthright to his brother Jacob he sold it in exchange for Jacob's red pottage or stew. There is a dish served in the Middle East to this day called Red Stew. It is made of beans and lentils boiled with garlic. It does not contain meat, but it undoubtedly smelled good to a hungry man:

> *Then Jacob gave Esau bread and pottage of lentils; and he did eat and drink, and rose up and went his way. (Genesis 25: 34)*

Does the Book of Mormon have anything to say? Yes. To cite just a few references, In I Nephi 8, Nephi records what his family gathered to take on their upcoming sea voyage:

> *And it came to pass that we had gathered together all manner of **seeds** of every kind, both of **grain** of every kind, and also of the seeds of **fruit** of every kind.*

They seem to have been in line with the advice we have today. Then in Alma 5 we see fruit and bread used as a metaphor for the best gifts just as they are in the Bible:

> Yea, he saith: Come unto me and ye shall partake of the **fruit** of the tree of life; yea, ye shall eat and drink of the **bread** and the waters of life freely.

As a final note here, it's interesting that the Lord lists grain, roots, and the fruit of the vine together. Do they have some characteristic in common? Whole grains and many roots including potatoes, sweet potatoes, yams, and beets as well as the vine crops, which include squashes and legumes are an excellent source of resistant starch.

What is resistant starch and why is it important? Resistant starches act on our digestion as a prebiotic, that is, foods with resistant starch feed the healthy microbes residing in our gut. Resistant starches are indigestible carbohydrates that pass through the small intestines into the large intestine where beneficial microbes feast on what they offer. It is different that fiber, but many of the plants high in resistant starches are also high in fiber, another prebiotic. There are gluten containing grains in this group. If gluten bothers you, don't choose those grains! There are plenty of others to choose from.

Don't overdo these foods. More is not better, but certainly have grains, roots and fruits of the vine daily.

EAT WHOLE GRAINS;

EAT THE FRUIT of THE VINE

and ROOTS.

7 IN SEASON

11 Every herb in the season thereof, and every fruit in the season thereof; *all these to be used with prudence and thanksgiving.*

What exactly does *in season* mean? I can't be sure what the Lord meant, but to me *in season* means in a fresh, natural or as close to a fresh and natural state as possible. Fresh fruits and vegetables in the state in which they grew are in season. However I don't think this means to only eat our fruits and vegetables raw or in the summertime. I am not a raw food advocate. Some vegetables actually release nutrients when cooked and are healthier than if eaten raw. Legumes are a good example of foods that need cooking—most people wouldn't think of making a meal of dry beans.

To me the phrase *in the season thereof* is a way of saying to avoid the highly processed foods that are available to us today. Why didn't the Lord speak to Joseph Smith more clearly? Couldn't he have said, "Avoid highly processed foods!" Maybe for the same reason the Lord said, "Hot drinks are not for the body or for the belly"? I don't think Joseph Smith or anyone else during his lifetime would have understood if the Lord had said, "Don't use hot drinks full of caffeine or acrylamide or tannins or whatever other problems there may be with coffee and tea. So He spoke in a language that could be understood at that time.

Of course fruits and vegetables were cooked and preserved at the time of Joseph Smith and even in biblical times. But the ability to preserve fruits and vegetables long term, let alone to transport fresh foods over long distances with refrigeration was rudimentary or non-existent at the time Joseph Smith received the Word of Wisdom. The processed foods that we have today were non-existent and unimaginable. Foods in the mid 1800s were preserved by drying, salting or fermenting, but they were not processed in the modern sense of the word. To advise eating foods in season, or in as natural a state as possible, was a no brainer in Joseph Smith's day, hardly necessary. This advice is there for us today with our plethora of processed foods.

Joseph Fielding Smith also felt the need to clarify this point. He explained, "Some have stumbled over the meaning of this expression and have argued that grains and fruits should only be used in the season of their growth and when they are ripened. This is not the intent, but any grain or fruit is out of season no matter what part of the year it may be if it is unfit for use." (16)

That brings us back to processed foods. What are processed foods? The Internet gives this definition: "Foods that are packaged in boxes, cans, or bags. These foods need to be processed extensively to be edible and are not found *as is in nature*." (17) For me processed foods, foods that are not found as in nature, are not *in season*.

My great grandfather Samuel Woolley left Nauvoo and headed west in 1847 in one of the first companies of Saints. He and his brother Edwin carried a barrel of dried apples in their wagon. Those apples, a source of vitamin C, kept their families safe from the ravages of black tongue or scurvy that afflicted many pioneer groups, including the Saints at Winter Quarters, during that first winter. Drying was a common form of food preservation along with salting and fermenting (think pickles). Dried apples can still be recognized as a food found in nature and are fit for use. They may even have saved lives for those who had them.

Canning was another step in food preservation. Canning is a relatively recent development and was not widely available until the mid to late nineteenth century. Canned goods are now available everywhere, and canning is a common practice in some homes. A woman asked me recently if she could be a good Latter-day Saint if she didn't like to can food. I told her emphatically, "Yes. Canning food is not an essential part of the gospel." Wow! There are many fruits and vegetables that can be canned successfully, but too often canning involves the addition not only of heat, but also of large amounts of sugar. Be careful how you preserve foods.

Freezing foods as a means of preservation prior to refrigeration (except inadvertently in the winter) was also nearly impossible. But freezing is an excellent method of food preservation today, maintaining many fruits and vegetables in a near fresh state. Most grocery stores' frozen fruits and vegetables are frozen at the farm, and have more nutrients than the "fresh" alternatives found in produce departments after their several days or weeks long trip to the store. But what we refer to as processed foods, foods with little resemblance to their natural counterparts, were fortunately unavailable at the time the Word of Wisdom was received.

The processed and refined foods available today are several steps away from *in season.* They are generally an unhealthy alternative to fresh foods, filled with sweeteners, heat processed oils, waxes and preservatives, food dyes, and chemicals. These processed products cannot be recognized as *foods found in nature.*

Think about sugar: Sugar is an ingredient in nearly all processed foods and is a highly processed food itself. Sugar is a plant extract, but it has no resemblance to the plant or even to the juice from which it originated, be it from sugar cane or sugar beets or corn or rice or any other sweet natural source. Most sweeteners are highly processed and are certainly not *in season* in any way. In fact, their highly processed forms are toxic to the body.

Consider carbonated or any other sugar or high fructose corn syrup sweetened drink. Read the label. These fizzy and not so fizzy drinks contain neither food sources nor nutritive value. Lemon lime flavoring. Extracts. Carmel coloring. Artificial coloring. Preservatives. They contain no natural food sources. No vitamins, no protein, no fat, no carbohydrates except sugars, no fiber—No nutritional value. What are you actually drinking? These drinks cannot be in season because they have no season. The same can be said for most, if not all, processed foods. We will talk more about sugars and processed and refined foods in later sections.

EAT ALL VEGETABLES and FRUITS IN SEASON.

Avoid Processed Foods

8 IS THAT ALL?

That's all folks! The Word of Wisdom is pretty simple. Many of the foods that are a part of our everyday diet aren't even mentioned in the Word of Wisdom. And of course that makes sense. Remember, God tells us:

It is not meet that I should command in all things. (Doctrine and Covenants 58: 26)

God doesn't command in all things and there are many things he has already told us in places other than the Word of Wisdom in the Doctrine and Covenants. We cannot and should not assume that just because something is not mentioned in the Word of Wisdom we shouldn't eat it. Common sense and a further reading of the scriptures will tell us there are healthy foods beyond those mentioned in section 89 of the Doctrine and Covenants.

For example, **water** is not mentioned in the Word of Wisdom. Whoa! Should we therefore not drink water?

Of course we should drink water. Water is essential to life.

Water is the most abundant compound on the surface of the earth. Every living creature, not just humans, needs water to live. Water is necessary for the functioning of our cells, tissues, and organs. Without water we would die. Remember, in Deuteronomy the Promised Land is described as having springs of clear water! Yet water is not mentioned anywhere in the Word of Wisdom.

Fish is not mentioned in the Word of Wisdom, nor is fish covered by the *category flesh of beast or fowls of the air.* We have already touched briefly on the importance of fish in the Bible, and nutritionally fish is a stellar food. Loaves and fishes were such a common meal in Biblical times that it comes as no surprise when Jesus refers to loaves and fishes various times in the New Testament. In the Sermon on the Mount Christ asks,

> *What man is there of you whom if his son ask bread, will give him a stone? Or if he ask a fish, will he give him a serpent? (Matthew 7: 9, 10)*

Why does Jesus use fish and bread as examples? Because, to make a comparison between good and evil gifts He used good and familiar foods. Jesus and His followers probably ate bread and fish every day, even for breakfast. (See John 21: 9)

I avoid meat or poultry, but I have added fish to my diet as a healthy source of animal protein. I've learned to cook and enjoy fish. Let me point out that in the nineteenth century in the United States, eggs, dairy, and fish were eaten in much greater quantities than we consume per capita today. There was no idea at that time that too many eggs might be harmful, or that dairy fats should be avoided if not eliminated completely from the diet. (Of course they skimmed off the fat for butter and cheese.) People worked hard. Their bodies needed the fat and proteins available in these foods, and so do we today.

But dairy products are not mentioned in the Word of Wisdom, nor are eggs, honey, nuts, or oils. What should we do about these important foods? Let's look at them one at a time starting with eggs. **Eggs** are referred to as a good gift in the Bible:

> *Which of you fathers, if your son asks for a fish, will give him a snake instead? OR if he asks for an egg, will give him a scorpion? If you then, though you are evil, know how to give good gifts to your children, how much more will your Father in heaven give the Holy Spirit to those who ask him! (Luke 11: 11-13)*

And what about dairy? **Milk** from both cows and goats was a readily available, and commonly used food in Biblical times:

> *. . . with curds and **milk** from herd and flock and with fattened lambs and goats, with choice rams of Bashan and the finest kernels of wheat. (Deuteronomy 32:14)*

The above verse refers to milk from both cattle and sheep or goats. Without refrigeration all types of milk had to be converted to butter and cheese, and yogurt or curds, which were easier to keep. There is another reference to milk in Isaiah 7: 21-22:

> In that day, a person will keep alive a young cow and two goats. And because of the abundance of the milk they give, there will be curds to eat. All who remain in the land will eat curds and honey.

Again, the term *curds* probably refers to yogurt. And who doesn't like yogurt with honey nowadays?

Without modern refrigeration, milk would have been purposely fermented to avoid spoilage. In addition to its preservative action fermentation adds live cultures, which can be beneficial to us. Natural yogurt and kefir are very nutritious. The bacterial cultures in these foods act as probiotics, improving and enhancing our gut flora, which we are learning is extremely important to nutrition, digestion and overall good health. Fermentation converts lactose or milk sugar to lactic acid, which is easier for many people to digest. Regardless, milk would have been converted to yogurt or used fresh. Skimmed butterfat would have been used to make butter and cheeses.

Many years ago my husband and I lived in a very rural area far from many of our modern conveniences and grocery stores. During that time I regularly bought raw milk from a neighbor. With my gallon of fresh milk I routinely skimmed off a portion of the cream, using it to make butter, sour cream, and whipped cream. Each gallon provided all the milk, butter, cream, and yogurt we ate. We did not buy a gallon of milk and then add additional butter and cream to the shopping cart. I always thought there was a kind of balance that we didn't maintain once we began buying our milk at the store. (I did not make cheese. I bought cheese at the cheese factory on our occasional trips into town.)

And speaking of cheeses, in I Samuel 17: 18, David's father instructs David to take ten cheeses to the commander of his brothers' military unit and bring back news. **Cheese** was a normal, healthy part of the diet in Biblical times.

In the book of Proverbs **butter** is used to make a funny comparison between apparently commonplace actions and the effects of anger:

> *For as churning cream produces butter, and as twisting the nose produces blood, so stirring up anger produces strife. (Proverbs 30:33)*

For those of you who have churned cream into butter the comparison with churning anger into strife is easy to understand. (Of course if you are lactose intolerant you will need to avoid fresh milk, but butter and yogurt contain less lactose than milk and may not cause the same digestive problems. Any healthy eating plan should be modified to avoid those foods that cause personal allergies or intolerances. Use common sense in what you choose to eat.)

Remember in the past everyone skimmed their milk. Milk proteins, whey and casein, are both beneficial to the biome and by extension to overall health. Milk sugar in moderation is also beneficial. But the saturated fat in milk affects the body in the same way that the saturated fats in meats do.

We know milk affects he biome positively and negatively. Larry Tucker, a professor at BYU, addressed the health implications of milk from a completely different angle. He studied how drinking milk affects our telomeres. Telomeres are the little end caps on our chromosomes. I visualize them somewhat like the little plasticized end on a shoelace. Anyway, our telomeres are closely correlated with aging. Every time a cell replicates itself the end cap or telomere shortens a tiny amount. The older we get the shorter our telomeres become.

Obviously some people age faster than others, some live longer. What kinds of things affect the health of our telomeres? According to Tucker, the more whole or 2% milk we drink, the shorter our telomeres become. Comparing adult whole milk drinkers with those who drank only non-fat milk, the whole milk drinkers' telomeres were 145 base pairs shorter than those of the non-fat milk drinkers. I don't know scientifically what exactly that means except that the non-fat milk drinkers were not aging as quickly as the whole milk drinkers. And as the body ages almost all systems are affected.

Should we stop drinking whole milk? Should we give up milk completely? Now this is really interesting. Tucker found that those who abstained from milk all together also had shorter telomeres than those who drank low or nonfat milk. So remember, going back to the studies on milk and the microbiome, milk proteins and even milk sugar has a beneficial affect on our microbiome and on our bodies. Don't give up milk. Just go easy on the cream and butter. Use low or non-fat milk.

Turning again to Biblical times, because butter turned rancid quickly and because it melted and burned at a fairly low temperature, a widely available alternative, olive oil, was most often used for cooking. **Olive oil** is not mentioned at all in the Word of Wisdom but it is mentioned often in the Bible as a food, as an ointment, and as a source of light. In Exodus 29: 2 the Israelites are instructed to make bread, cakes and wafers using fine wheat flour and olive oil. And when Elijah asks a widow woman to make him something to eat she tells him she has only enough flour and olive oil for a small meal for herself and her son before they starve to death:

> *And she said, as the LORD thy God liveth, I have not a cake, but an handful of meal in a barrel, and a little oil in a cruse: and, behold, I am gathering two*

sticks, that I may go in and dress it for me and my
son, that we may eat it, and die. (1 Kings 17:12)

Pretty grim, but instead of feeding herself and her son, the woman makes a cake for the prophet, and her flour and oil last her thereafter for many days.

Before we continue I want to say just a little bit more about oil. Think how much better Elijah's little cake must have tasted with the addition of oil, rather than just flour and water. It would have had a better texture as well as taste. But many people today believe the less oil or fat we consume the better. Health wise this is completely untrue. We need fats and oils in our diets and we need them every day. And the fat we need the most is an essential fatty acid classified as omega-3 fatty acid.

Our brain is sixty percent fat, (yep, that's true.) and omega-3 fatty acids make up almost half of that fat in the brain. So omega-3 fatty acids make up nearly 30% of our total brain. Our bodies cannot build omega-3 fatty acids by recombining other sources of fat. Omega-3 fatty acids are an essential fatty acid, or in other words a fatty acid that must be consumed to be available in the body. Without this fatty acid neither the body nor the brain can function at an optimal level.

Where do we get omega-3 fatty acids since our bodies cannot produce them from other sources? Let me say again, omega-3 fatty acid is an essential fatty acid, one that has to be ingested, eaten from foods containing omega-3 fatty acids. We need this fatty acid; it is essential to our health and well-being; it is essential to our brain. And where is the best place to get omega-3 fatty acid?

Olive Oil is a moderately good source of this fatty acid, but not the best source. Olive oil does contain both Omega 3 and Omega 6 fatty acids. These two fatty acids work in concert and we feel the best when they are balanced in our bodies. The ratio of these two fatty acids in the diet is extremely important, as they can enhance or inhibit one another. The ratio of omega-3s to omega-6s is very good in olive oil. (Heat processing on the other hand, destroys the omega-3 fatty acids in almost all grocery store vegetable oils, leaving a very unhealthy ratio of inflammation-causing omega-6 fatty acids alone.) (18)

But, however good olive oil is for us, the best source of omega-3 fatty acids is FISH. Fish oil is our number one source of this important brain food. Omega-3 fatty acids are of primary importance in maintaining the structure and function of the brain. In other words our brains need omega-3 fatty acids to function properly. Omega-3 fatty acids facilitate communication between brain cells. As nerve impulses pass from one neuron to another they must be able to get through the membrane surrounding that neuron. Omega-3 fatty acids make this transmission possible. Omega-3s also increase the production of vital neurotransmitters; those important feel-good chemicals that help us control our moods. Omega-3s reduce oxidation and inflammation (19) in the brain after an injury.

We need omega-3 fatty acids, and we need a specific form, DHA. DHA is one of several variations of omega-3s, and it accounts for 97% of the omega-3s found in the brain. DHA is a major structural component of the cerebral cortex, the area of the brain responsible for memory, creativity, emotion, and attention. People with low levels of DHA have measurably smaller brains than normal. (20) Ever wonder why you have memory problems or attention problems? Feed your brain! Another important form of omega-3 fatty acid is EPA. EPA promotes healthy blood flow to the brain and so keeps us sharp.

Omega-3 fatty acids accumulate in the fetal brain during development. It is crucial for brain growth and development from the embryonic state through birth, continuing in the developing infant. (21) Developing embryos have to get those vital Omega-3s from their mothers. On the other side of life, when levels of omega-3 fatty acids are low aging is accelerated and deficits in brain function occur, increasing the risk of dementia, schizophrenia and Alzheimer's disease. Eat more fish.

Remember, your body cannot make omega-3 fatty acids. You have to get them in your diet. You need them, your children need them, even your unborn children need them. Children whose mothers take fish oil supplements during pregnancy have higher intellectual ability and better social skills than their peers and are less likely to develop ADHD, autism or cerebral palsy, and omega-3 fatty acids have been found to be helpful in the treatment of major depressive disorders. I read recently that omega-3 fatty acids have not proven to be useful in prevention of heart disease. Oh well. Think about how important this nutrient is and don't worry that it doesn't solve every physical problem around!

But why am I suddenly taking so much time to talk about a specific nutrient? Because I know that many of you think you don't like fish. And even more of you may think that a healthy diet is a very low-fat diet. We need fat and oil and fish to stay healthy. Fish and seafood are the richest sources of omega-3 fatty acids available to us. A serving of fish provides many times the amount of fish oil you'll get in a fish oil capsule and it is likely to be fresher and more digestible. Try fish. Add fish to your daily or weekly meals. (Fish is also and excellent source of vitamin B12, for those who are not eating other meats. B12 is only accessible from animal sources. True vegetarians are counseled to take a B12 supplement regularly.)

Add and enjoy fats and oils. Our bodies need a number of essential oils. Fish oil with its omega-3 fatty acids is just one, but it is a very important one. Later we'll talk more about olive oils and other healthy oils. Don't overdo it, but don't avoid fats and oils either. Remember Christ ate fish and olive oil every day. They are good for you too.

What else should we consider? Ezekiel compared

Jerusalem to a beautiful woman who has received all the finest things in life including fine flour, honey and oil:

> *Thus wast thou decked with gold and silver; and thy raiment was of fine linen, and silk, and broidered work; thou didst eat fine flour, and honey, and oil: and thou wast exceeding beautiful, and thou didst prosper into a kingdom. (Ezekiel 16:13)*

Honey and oil add to and enhance the flavor and nutritive value of food. They are not only delicious they are beneficial. Proverbs 16 tells just how beneficial **honey** is:

> *Pleasant words are a honeycomb, Sweet to the soul and healing to the bones. (Proverbs 16:24)*

In 1 Samuel Jonathan, son of Saul, remarks:

> *See how my eyes have brightened because I tasted a little of this honey. (1 Samuel 14: 29)*

Even Isaiah mentions honey:

> *Butter and honey shall he eat, that he may know to refuse the evil, and choose the good.*
> *(Isaiah 7: 15)*

I recently saw an interpretation of this scripture that equated butter to evil and honey to good. I believe that butter and honey in this reference are both good and having once tasted the good we can reject what is not good. And don't forget the Promised Land, a land flowing with milk and honey, which implies a good land with plenty of water in order to support blossoms and grassy fields where cattle, goats and bees all thrive.

Finally, in Proverbs we are told:

> My son, eat honey, for it is good, Yes, the honey from the comb is sweet to your taste. (Proverbs 24: 13).

But Proverbs goes on to warn against eating too much honey. I guess we can get too much of a good thing. So let's not overdo it.

> Hast thou found honey? Eat so much as is sufficient for thee, lest thou be filled therewith, and vomit. (Proverbs 25: 16)

Finally, from the Book of Mormon:

> And they did also carry with them **Deseret**, which, by interpretation, is a honey bee; and thus they did carry with them swarms of bees, and all manner of that which was upon the face of the land and seeds of every kind. (Ether 2:3)

I imagine Deseret as the queen bee, (perhaps carried separately from the hive in a box) so that the swarm would follow. And I have also wondered how it was traveling across the ocean in a closed vessel with a swarm of bees! Certainly honey must be an important and nutritious addition to our diet (and to pollination) to warrant carrying the bees so far.

There would have already been bees in the Promised Land by the time Lehi's family arrived. But in 1 Nephi: 18: 6 we see that Lehi's family also carried honey:

> *And it came to pass that on the morrow, after we had prepared all things, much fruits and meat from the wilderness, and honey in abundance, and provisions according to that which the Lord had commanded us, we did go down into the ship, with all our loading and our seeds, and whatsoever thing we had brought with us, every one according to his age; wherefore, we did all go down into the ship, with our wives and our children.*

And yes, they carried honey in abundance. Interestingly only honey and pure maple sugar are gut friendly sweeteners, both to be used in moderation.

There are many healthy, nutritious foods not mentioned in the Word of Wisdom, foods that add flavor and substance to our meals. Even **spices** add important phytonutrients and are one of our best sources of antioxidants. Jacob refers to some of these in the Bible calling them some of the best products of the land.

> *Then their father Israel said to them, "If it must be, then do this: Put some of the best products of the land in your bags and take them down to the man as a gift—a little balm and a little honey, some*

*spices and myrrh, some pistachio **nuts** and almonds. (Genesis 43: 11)*

Here's where we are so far:

HONEY, NUTS, SPICES

HEALTHY OILS

MILK and YOGURT

CHEESE and EGGS

VINES AND ROOTS

GRAINS

FISH

LEAFY GREENS AND FRUITS

(Leafy greens and fruit are the foundation of good health.)

IMPLEMENTATION

9 STEP 1: LEAFY GREENS

(Try to follow each step for at least a week. If you feel like you need more time, stick with that step for a second week or as long as you need to feel comfortable and successful with it.)

Before we start getting rid of things and emptying the cupboards let's add something delicious to the foods we normally eat. And let's imagine the bounty the Word of Wisdom offers. Imagine your dining room table: places are set for the family, and the center of the table is filled with serving dishes and platters. There are bowls filled with seeds and nuts, platters filled with well seasoned fish, soufflés, sautéed vegetables, fruits, soups, spicy chili beans, fruit salads, strawberries and yogurt, green salads with olive oil dressing, cheeses of all types, crunchy breads. Okay, that's too much for one meal. But this is how you can and should be planning. Keep this picture in mind as we build step by step toward a new way of eating.

The Word of Wisdom starts off with leafy greens, vegetables and fruits. Let's start by adding two to four or more cups of greens to what we eat everyday and at least one serving of fruit. It shouldn't be too hard to do. There are nearly 1,100 different vegetables in the world and nearly 500 of those are leafy vegetables. We have plenty to choose from!

 Of course the easiest way to add greens is to make a salad. Maybe you eat salads already. If you do, expand and eat more. Use cruciferous vegetables like kale and cabbage and cauliflower and broccoli. Use and celery and carrots and cilantro and lots of kinds of lettuce and spinach, romaine lettuce, collard greens, mustard greens, bok choy, turnip greens and watercress and beets and apples and blueberries and—you know what you like in a salad. So make a big salad and eat it every day even if it doesn't have all that variety.

Or, you can choose to cook cabbage or broccoli or cauliflower plain or in a soup. Or make a spinach smoothie. This week eat greens everyday. And eat fruit—fresh fruit— every day. You can eat an orange or a nectarine in place of your morning orange juice. You can throw berries into your smoothie. One serving of fruit a day is easy. Have more if you want to.

I often have a big salad for lunch. I buy a bag of chopped greens, pour two or three cupsful into a bowl, add a scoop of cottage cheese as dressing, cut up and add strawberries or apples, and top it off with a can of tuna. It's a big salad. It is probably my biggest meal of the day by volume and I always enjoy it.

But don't worry about the tuna yet. The tuna in that salad will carry us over to step two.

Did I have 2 to 4 cups of leafy greens today and at least one serving of fruit?

Step 1	M	T	W	Th	Fr	S	Su
Greens							
Fruit							

How did your week go? Are you ready to move on?

10 STEP 2: FISH

After leafy greens and fruit the Word of Wisdom goes right to meat and poultry. And it tells us NOT to eat the flesh of beasts or fowls that walk, run, crawl, or fly over the earth. This week we will add fish to the diet. It swims in the water. No flying, no creeping. And it has been an important part of the human diet for millennia. Only recently has fish fallen out of favor as an everyday food.

During week two and three transition from meat and chicken to eating only fish as your source of animal protein during at least one meal at least three days a week. (Well you can still have eggs and dairy. Fish will be your only meat.)

Fish is very nutritious. It's good for you. And it is surprisingly tasty. You might have to figure out how to cook it to your taste. But that's what this step is for. During at least three meals this week try fish. Tuna may be the most familiar fish in your pantry. And tuna is a fairly healthy fish. Start with tuna if you'd like. (Normally I eat fish between four and five times a week. I don't necessarily feel like I need animal protein every day. Maybe you won't either.)

Maybe you wonder why, if the Lord counsels us against the flesh of beasts and fowls, we would need any animal protein. Good question. Protein is made up of amino acids and amino acids are the essential building blocks of our bodies—our skin, bones, muscles, hair and fingernails, and even our DNA and the neurotransmitters that help control mood.

Feeling depressed? Maybe you need to eat a little fish. Or eggs. Of course beans also contain a fair amount of protein and are an excellent addition to the diet. We'll talk more about beans later, but fish and eggs give us a more complete protein than we get from most plant proteins. Both fish and eggs contain all of the important and essential amino acids our bodies need. And fish is also the best source of the omeaga-3 fatty acids that we need— you'd have to eat a lot of walnuts to match fish. Beans are a good source of protein, but not as good for fatty acids.

It may be easier to implement this step over a two week period. During the first week try to eliminate red meat, and continue to eat the leafy greens and fruit from step one. During the next week let go of chicken and fowl. Both weeks add fish. You can easily add fish to your salads, or make a tuna sandwich. But I recommend that you try to add fish at least three days this week as your dinner entrée.

WEEK 2

1. Did I have 2 to 3 cups of leafy greens today and at least one serving of fruit?
2. Did I add fish several days this week? Did I eliminate red meat this week?

Step 1	M	T	W	Th	F	S	Su
Greens							
Fruit							
Step 2							
Fish							

WEEK 3

1. Did I have 2 to 3 cups of leafy greens today and at least one serving of fruit?
2. Did I add fish several days this week? Did I eliminate chicken this week?

Step 1	M	T	W	Th	F	S	Su
Greens							
Fruit							
Step 2							
Fish							

Are you ready for step 3?

11 STEP 3: GRAINS

As you begin Step 3 remember to continue eating two to four cups of leafy greens daily, and continue eating fish 3 or 4 days a week, eliminating meat and poultry.

This week let's take on whole grains and breakfast. There is a full complement of healthy grains to choose from but the best known and most commonly consumed are wheat and oats. But before we look at wheat and oats let's take all your processed cereals out of the kitchen.

Most breakfast cereals aren't whole grain and they are definitely not healthy. Many breakfast cereals are candy in disguise, highly processed, high in sugar and preservatives, low in nutrients, and very bad for breakfast. They're easy but they're not good. They're not good for you and they're not a healthy start to the day for your kids. Luckily we've been given a much better alternative in whole grains.

Starting on day one this week replace your cereal boxes with whole grain cereals. Oatmeal, rolled oats, steel cut oats, whole grain, low-sugar granola (you really have to check labels or make your own granola) shredded wheat, cream of wheat, whole or cracked wheat cooked in the crock-pot. Wheat and oats are only two of countless grains. You can continue this list with barley and rye, and any other grains you choose.

This week replace cold, boxed cereal with whole grain cereals.

Next goes white bread. Take it out of the house. When you make toast use breads that say whole wheat or whole grain on the label. Whole wheat should be first on the ingredient list and there should be no white flour or wheat flour on the list. (You could make your own whole grain bread.)

Be careful, even when the label says whole wheat it may not be 100% whole wheat; but it will be better than the bread that doesn't say whole wheat at all. And if the label lists *wheat flour* or *wheat bread* it absolutely is not whole wheat bread. *Wheat flour* on the label always refers to refined white flour. Darn it! And that brown colored bread that says wheat bread? Yes, it is made with refined white flour with caramel coloring added. You don't have to believe me, read the labels.

Why are we throwing out the white bread? I for one don't believe the Word of Wisdom is referring to white flour when it talks positively about wheat and other grains. I'm pretty sure that the Word of Wisdom refers to whole grains and whole grain flours. Why?

First, white flour wasn't available on a large scale until after 1845, and it was virtually unavailable to all but the very wealthy at the time the Word of Wisdom was received. Two hundred years ago the average human everywhere on the earth ate hardly any white flour in a lifetime and less than ten pounds of sugar in an entire year—not even a pound a month. Things changed in the 1890s as the craze for carbonated cola drinks swept across the United States and then the world. If you were thirsty and needed a drink, you could suddenly, fashionably drink sugar water—carbonated sugar water.

In that same decade mills capable of refining wheat into white flour at a reasonable price (producing flour devoid of any nutritional value) were developed and suddenly nearly everybody could afford white flour. Only after people became ill did the mills start "enriching" their flour with a handful of the vitamins that had been removed. Yet for some reason everybody still wanted that fancy, nutrition-free flour.

But that was later, well after the Mormon pioneers' migration to Utah. The pioneers carried and used whole wheat flour as they crossed the plains. The idea of refining flour, removing the fiber, the germ and the vitamins and sometimes bleaching what was left over, would never have occurred to the pioneers for whom bread formed a substantial part of their daily diet and filled many of their nutritional needs.

For most of history bread, the most important staple food in the world was made using whole wheat flour. When the poor widow in the Bible made a cake for the prophet Elijah with oil and fine flour, she was using fine whole wheat flour. When Christ increased the loaves and fishes his disciples had collected to feed the five thousand, he was working with whole wheat bread. People in the nineteenth century took it for granted that flour was by definition whole wheat flour.

Second, once you've taken away the fiber or bran, the germ, the vitamins and the minerals it's hard to think of white flour as an *in season grain*. White flour is deficient nutritionally. If it weren't enriched it would not sustain life. But why take out the naturally occurring vitamins, fiber and other nutrients and then add back only a handful of synthetic vitamins and try to convince me that you've improved the product? I think white flour should be used sparingly, maybe as a condiment. It works for thickening gravy for example. But otherwise it is not the staff of life.

I have tried many recipes for homemade whole wheat bread, not all successful. I finally have a recipe I like. But there are good breads available at the grocery store. Try not to make this too difficult! Read labels. Buy good bread.

So this week we're replacing processed breakfast cereals with whole grains, and breads made with refined flour with whole- wheat/whole grain breads.

Focus on breakfast this week and then expand your whole grains to cover the rest of the day—any bread or grains you have at lunch and dinner. If you need more time, take more time. And at Step 4 we'll only add good foods without taking anything away.

Remember grains and cereals are feeding your gut biome. Eat and enjoy these foods!

1. Did I have 2 to 3 cups of leafy greens today and at least one serving of fruit?
2. Did I add fish several days this week? Did I eliminate other meats?
3. Did I eat whole grains for breakfast? Am I only using whole grain breads?

Step 1	M	T	W	Th	F	S	Su
Greens							
Fruit							
Step 2							
Fish							
Step 3							
Breads							
Cereal							

Are you ready for step 4?

12 STEP 4: VINES AND ROOTS

This week we'll add more fruits and vegetables, fresh or frozen. This is the week for vines and roots. Vines and roots along with whole grains give us resistant starches and a healthy gut. What is resistant starch? Resistant starches are just what the name implies. They are not easily broken down and digested in the stomach, nor in the small intestine. They travel all the way to the large intestine where they feed the good bacteria and fungi there and help in the synthesis of enzymes, vitamins and other nutrients. Grains, potatoes, winter squash, legumes, and more all contain resistant starch. It's interesting that these foods are mentioned together, almost as a separate category in the Word of Wisdom. I guess that's how important they are to our health.

So, here come potatoes, and yams and beets, peas and beans and whole grains. And that's not all. Berries and melons and cucumbers and summer squash and carrots, onions and garlic, and grapes and—well you can make your own list—are all filled with phytonutrients and antioxidants and are important for our health. These vegetables and fruits will not only enhance your oatmeal, they'll make your smoothies better, they'll fill out your lunches, dinners and snacks, and they'll make great desserts. So add these fresh fruits and vegetables at every meal.

Oh, and don't forget legumes. Legumes are almost in a class by themselves. Besides containing resistant starch they're a great source of protein. Beans? I could eat beans everyday. Some mornings I have beans with my eggs for breakfast. Sometimes I add beans to my salads. I make chili, and bean stew, and bean soup. Of course legumes are more than just beans. And legumes are one of the healthiest, most delicious foods available.

How healthy? Consider this: One hundred grams of beef and 100 grams of pinto beans each have 22 grams of protein. That's right, the beans have the same amount of protein as the steak. But beans also have 15 grams of fiber. Meat contains no fiber. Fiber is only found in plant foods. The steak has almost 2 milligrams of iron; the beans have 5 milligrams of iron. The steak provides 16 mg of calcium and 23 mg of magnesium; but the beans provide 123 mg of calcium and 171 mg of magnesium. Bite for bite the beans are the healthier choice. And protein is metabolized more slowly and is therefore more available to the body when it is eaten with fiber. Beans win again!

Do you make your chili with hamburger or with sirloin steak? Try it in step five without the meat or cut the amount of meat you were using previously in half. Think of meat as a seasoning. Very little will do the trick and your chili, etc. will still taste really good. One step at a time, one meal at a time continue to modify your diet keeping the Word of Wisdom and excellent health squarely in mind. Add beans, peas, peanuts, and lentils to your meals as a side dish or a main course.

Remember Daniel and his diet of pulse (legumes) and water. Eat beans and be ten times better! These foods also feed your gut. As Daniel found out, they are super foods!

1.Did I have 2 to 4 cups of leafy greens today and at least one serving of fruit?
2. Did I add fish several days this week?
3.Did I eat whole grains for breakfast? Am I only using whole grain breads?
4.Have I added root and vine fruits and vegetables? Did I eat legumes at least once a week?

Step 1	M	T	W	Th	F	S	Su
Greens							
Fruit							
Step 2							
Fish							

Step 3						
Breads						
Cereal						
Step 4						
Vines						
Roots						
Legumes						

13 STEP 5: IN SEASON

If you have been following the steps in this program you have now spent a month or more working to change and modify what you eat. What and how we eat is one of our most basic activities. It can be hard to make changes at this level. But you have been working at it in the hopes of living not only a healthier and more abundant life but also a life more in keeping with the plan the Lord has offered us. These are worthy goals. So let's pause and review.

You are now eating lots of green leafy vegetables everyday along with some fruit. You have cut meat from your regular diet and perhaps added fish. You are eating whole grains for breakfast, maybe with fresh fruit and without sugar, and you're eating whole grain breads during the day. You are trying out new and creative recipes with legumes as well as other vine and root vegetables and fruits.

As you follow this plan you are leaving behind the typical American diet.

What is the typical American diet?

Well, I'll just say it's not good. The three most consumed foods in America are white bread, coffee, and hotdogs. Go ahead and cross coffee off that list. You were evidently somewhat atypical already! And now white bread and hot dogs are gone! That was lucky. The typical American diet is making us all unhealthy and overweight.

Let's look at processed foods and some of the problems they present. Processed foods are obviously a major part of the typical American diet, and processed foods are high in sweeteners, white flour, heat-processed oils, salt, preservatives, additives, and artificial coloring. None of these ingredients are natural or nutritious or in season. Processed foods are lacking in the healthy, nutritious ingredients that allow us to run and not be weary and walk and not faint. Processed foods are low in overall nutritional value. They don't usually contain much protein and they contain no healthy fats, no complex carbohydrates, and little or no fiber. They are lacking in vitamins and minerals. What they do have is a high sugar content and a high percentage of heat-processed, unhealthy oils. Processed foods provide little in the way of nutrition other that added calories. They do contain calories, plenty of calories, many of them from sugars.

How much sugar do we consume per capita? Too much. To compare, in 1828 people ate about twelve pounds of sugar and other caloric sweeteners (think maple syrup, honey, etc.) per year or about a pound a month. Diabetes was nearly unknown. In fact, diabetes was so rare that doctors might treat one or two cases in the course of their entire professional careers. But by 1963 20% of total daily calories and nearly half our carbohydrates were in the form of sugars. And it gets worse: In the mid '70s with the introduction of high fructose corn syrup our sugar consumption took a great leap forward bringing a corresponding increase in the rates of diabetes and obesity. By 1975 individual Americans were consuming 124 pounds of caloric sweeteners per year. (I use the term sugar or caloric sweeteners here to refer to all caloric sweeteners—sucrose, corn syrup, high fructose corn syrup, and any of the other caloric sweeteners.) By 1999 that number had risen to 158 pounds—nearly a half a pound of sugars each and every day for every man, woman, and child in the United States. (21) This adds up to a daily intake of about 750 calories per person from sugars. Sugars, which are nutrient free, may make up one third or more of the calories an average adult American consumes every a day.

The United States government recommends adults consume 300 grams of carbohydrates daily. At the consumption level shown above sugars account for 190 of the 300 grams of our daily carbohydrate allowance. So sugars make up 60% or more of total daily carbohydrate consumption—more than half! —as recommended by the government and enjoyed by the average American. And as used here, carbohydrates refer not only to the simple carbs in sugars and white flour, but to fruits, grains, vegetables and legumes, which should be the main source of our carbohydrate grams.

Except for salt, which is an essential nutrient and a naturally occurring mineral, sugar is the only pure crystal humans consume as a food. Sugar is an extract from plant sources but has been so highly processed there is no nutritional value remaining in the sweet-tasting, artificial crystal we eat. Sugar has no nutritional value. None. No vitamins, no minerals, no antioxidants. It provides calories and nothing else.

But what is the matter with eating a sweet non-nutrient, really? Is it enough of a reason to avoid sugar just because it is highly processed? What does sugar do in the body? Before I begin let me repeat: I am using the word sugar to refer to all caloric sweeteners: sucrose, cane sugar, brown sugar, white sugar, molasses, agave syrup, fructose, high fructose corn syrup—all sweeteners that contain calories. Non-caloric sweeteners are a different category and have problems of their own, but are probably no less damaging to our health than sugars.

The nutritious complex carbohydrates we eat are broken down and enter the bloodstream as glucose, a simple sugar and a component of all caloric sweeteners. Glucose is the body's primary source of energy providing energy or fuel directly to our muscles, cells, brain and other tissues. Excess glucose is converted to glycogen and stored in our muscles and liver as a future energy source. But even though all carbs break down into glucose, all carbs are not the same. Sugars or caloric sweeteners have properties that set them apart from more complex carbohydrates.

Sucrose, the chemical name for cane sugar, table sugar, brown sugar, and any other products made from sugar cane or sugar beets, consists of a molecule of fructose chemically bound to a molecule of glucose. Because the molecules are bound together, sucrose cannot be broken down in the stomach and so does not enter the bloodstream directly. In the small intestine the enzyme sucrase unlocks the glucose/fructose bond and releases two separate simple sugars. Once the sucrose bond is opened the fructose molecule travels from the small intestine into the liver while the glucose molecule moves into the bloodstream. Once in the bloodstream glucose is used for energy or stored as glycogen depending on the needs of our muscles and other cells. Fructose has bypassed the bloodstream and will likely never make it into the bloodstream to be used as a source of energy. Instead fructose is converted to fat by the liver and sent to storage in the fat cells.

Honey is similar to sucrose in many ways. It is made up of a molecule of glucose and a molecule of fructose. But the glucose and fructose in honey are not bound together, so the glucose separates from the fructose in the stomach and enters the bloodstream directly. Fructose is still metabolized in the small intestine and sent to the liver to be stored as a future energy source. But honey contains some vitamins and minerals and some digestive enzymes provided by the bee that help break it down in digestion. Honey (and maple syrup)in limited amounts actually has a positive effect on the gut.

High fructose corn syrup is made up of 55% or more fructose and 45% or less glucose. As with honey the glucose in high fructose corn syrup is metabolized directly from the stomach while the fructose travels to the small intestine and is redirected to the liver. Despite the labeling high fructose corn syrup can be as high as eighty-five percent fructose. So the glucose enters and saturates the bloodstream as a source of energy while a huge amount of fructose is sent to the liver and on to storage. This helps explain why obesity and type II diabetes rates rose along with the increased use of high fructose corn syrup in soft drinks beginning in the 1970s.

None of these sweeteners is healthy or necessary. Walter Glinsmann, author of a report on sugar for the United States Food and Drug Administration, labeled sucrose "the most lipogenic of carbohydrates"—or in other words the most fat producing. (22) Unfortunately high fructose corn syrup has replaced sucrose as the most lipogenic carbohydrate, and because high fructose corn syrup is slightly sweeter than sucrose and the most liquid-soluble sweetener it has become the sweetener of choice for soft drinks.

None of these highly processed sweeteners are good for us. Worse, they are directly harmful. The problem with fructose is not just weight gain, which we may not like, but also the accompanying diseases including insulin resistance, diabetes, heart disease, and high blood pressure. All of these diseases are linked to consumption of sugars. And so is tooth decay. For people who are not overweight, but who suffer from these health conditions, sugars are the most likely culprit or at least a contributing factor. When God said to eat foods in season He was concerned for our well-being. He wants us to be well nourished, healthy and feel good. He wants us to live a long and functional life.

A side note here on caffeine: Caffeine has been found in some studies to decrease insulin sensitivity, or in other words, caffeine may increase insulin resistance. Combine caffeine with the sugar in soft drinks, coffee and tea, and you have a potentially dangerous combination that can lead to or exacerbate type II diabetes or pre-diabetes. Caffeine combined with sugar may give you a double whammy health wise. Maybe that's why we were told to avoid those hot drinks—coffee and tea. What we do with the cold ones is up to us. But we should use wisdom.

Should we avoid carbs? Only simple carbs. Those healthy herbs, vegetables, and fruits are all complex carbohydrates. When I think of a high carbohydrate diet I don't usually think of a diet high in sugar, but sugars currently account for 60% or more of carbohydrate consumption in the typical American diet. And at the typical American grocery store we can only avoid sugars by conscientious choice and effort. The Word of Wisdom does not endorse a diet in which more than half our carbohydrates come from sugars. It's not healthy and it's not centered on natural leafy greens, fruits, vines, and roots in season.

Not surprisingly the top nutrient rich foods, the natural foods we should be eating, tend to be low in calories and high in vitamins, minerals, antioxidants, fiber, proteins, fats, and carbohydrates, just the opposite of processed foods. A list of the top mineral rich foods includes nuts and seeds, lentils and beans, dark leafy green vegetables, fish and shellfish, mushrooms, whole grains, milk and yogurt, avocados, dark chocolate, cheese, and dried fruit. Not surprisingly these are the very foods suggested in the Word of Wisdom and other scriptures. We need nutrient rich foods.

This week conscientiously read labels and select foods in their natural or near natural state. (For me that is pretty much fresh, dried, or frozen fruits and vegetables, whole and milled grains including whole grain flours, and fresh or frozen fish.

This week may call for some of the biggest changes in

what you eat so far. Instead of just making healthy additions to your diet, you may need to eliminate some of your old favorites and standbys. This week eliminate sugars and all products that contain sugars from your kitchen, from your desk, and from your car. Good-bye candy bars!

This week select and eat foods without added sugars, preservatives or other signs of over processing. One good rule of thumb is *Don't eat anything in a box or bag that contains more than three ingredients.* Read labels. Most of the time this will be a good guideline for shopping.

1. Did I have 2 to 3 cups of leafy greens today and at least one serving of fruit?
2. Did I add fish several days this week?
3. Did I eat whole grains for breakfast? Am I only using whole grain breads?
4. Have I added root and vine fruits and vegetables? Did I eat legumes at least once this week?
5. Did I eliminate processed foods morning, noon, and night?

Step 1	M	T	W	Th	F	S	Su
Greens							
Fruit							
Step 2							
Fish							
Step 3							
Breads							
Cereal							
Step 4							
Vines							
Roots							
Legumes							
Step 5							
No process							

Am I ready for Step 6?

14 STEP 6: DAIRY AND EGGS

By now you have added the core foods mentioned in the Word of Wisdom to your diet. Let's fill it out a little with some of the extras. It's time to add dairy and eggs. Milk, yogurt, cheese, and eggs were a part of the typical diet in Biblical times, and are all mentioned in the Bible as healthy and nutritious additions to the diet. They can and should be a healthy addition to our diet today. (If you are lactose intolerant skip milk. But butter, cheese and yogurt should be okay. Of course common sense suggests that you skip any foods you have an allergy or intolerance to.)

Eggs have had a bad reputation for many years, but eggs are a healthy source of protein and fat as well as an excellent source of vitamins and minerals. And we now know that eating eggs is not what raises cholesterol levels. Besides providing nutrients eggs help strengthen the immune system. As an excellent source of choline they improve memory and responsiveness. As a source of vitamin D eggs may help combat depression and strengthen teeth and bones. The protein in eggs does wonders for the fingernails and hair as well as other tissues. And finally, researchers in China have discovered a clear connection between eggs and a *reduced* risk of cardiovascular diseases—just the opposite of what we were told about eggs for years! (22)

So this week have eggs for breakfast, scrambled, fried or poached! Make a quiche, make a frittata, have an omelette (filled with spinach of course!). Enjoy eggs with any or every meal.

And don't forget dairy. Dairy has also gotten a bad rap for too long. Only yogurt seemed to survive the slamming of dairy's reputation. Yogurt is a very good form of milk as long as you make it with low or non-fat milk and don't load it up with sugars. The fermentation of milk into yogurt is beneficial to the good bacteria in our intestinal tract. Our gut bacteria help digest our food so we need to keep them well fed.

Dr. Ghannoum, a top researcher in the ongoing mapping of our intestinal biome, discovered to his surprise that people who severely limit their dairy intake following what is widely considered an extremely healthy diet are likely to experience digestive health symptoms such as bloating and intestinal upset. By cutting out dairy people may be inadvertently allowing aggressive intestinal fungi to grow out of balance. (23) Both the proteins and the carbohydrates in milk support the growth of good bacteria and fungi and help suppress negative microbes in the digestive tract. When we cut out dairy we cut out a support for the good bacteria and fungi in the gut. Dr. Ghannoum goes so far as to say, skip the cookies but drink the milk. While sugar can have a detrimental affect of the microbiome, lactose or milk sugar seems to be particularly beneficial even causing changes that are helpful to people with irritable bowel syndrome.

Good sources of dairy include low or non-fat milk, cottage cheese, kefir milk, and low-fat yogurt. Butter, and cheese should be used in moderation. If you are lactose intolerant you may still be able to enjoy fermented forms of dairy—kefir, yogurt and some cheeses—since lactose, the milk sugar or carbohydrate component of milk, is broken down during fermentation. Low fat and nonfat dairy is the best.

This week add dairy to your meals. Drink milk if you like it. Add low-fat grated cheeses to your vegetables and beans. Make smoothies with berries and plain low-fat yogurt. Add yogurt and eggs to your bread recipes. There are so many delicious ways to add eggs and dairy to your day. Just remember to continue with your greens and fruit, fish, grains, roots and vines. And while you're at it have a string cheese with that bunch of grapes or an omelet for breakfast. Delicious.

1. Did I have 2 to 4 cups of leafy greens today and at least one serving of fruit?

2. Did I add fish several days this week?
3. Did I eat whole grains for breakfast? Am I only using whole grain breads?
4. Have I added root and vine fruits and vegetables? Did I eat legumes at least once this week?
5. Have I eliminated processed foods?
6. Have I added eggs and low fat dairy to enhance my diet?

Step 1	M	T	W	Th	F	S	Su
Greens							
Fruit							
Step 2							
Fish							
Step 3							
Breads							
Cereal							
Step 4							
Vines							
Roots							
Legumes							
Step 5							
No process							
Step 6							
Eggs							
Dairy							

Am I ready for Step 7?

15   STEP 7: HONEY, OILS, NUTS, SEEDS AND SPICES

We talked about honey briefly in Chapter 13. **Honey** is the best natural, unprocessed sweetener we have. Honey was eaten and enjoyed in Biblical times but the amount of honey available in the everyday diet was tiny compared to the amounts of sugars we consume today. I use honey in cooking, but because of honey's unique properties I find that I can't use honey like I would sugar. I don't use a lot of honey, but I enjoy it when I do.

This week continue to limit your use of sweeteners, but if you do want something sweet use honey in place of other caloric sweeteners. The recipes in this book use honey in place of sugar and I have provided equivalent measurements in the back.

This week also be aware of the oils you use and make changes where needed. The first big change is to stop being afraid to use fats and oils in your daily diet. The low-fat craze that lasted for more than fifty years was accompanied by record rates of obesity and diabetes, and it didn't lower the rates of heart disease and hypertension. Ironic isn't it? Our bodies and our brains need fat. Complex carbohydrates eaten with fiber, fat, or protein enter the blood stream at a slower rate and cause less impact on blood sugar. That's the way the body works, and that's the way we're supposed to eat. Regardless, the carbohydrates we eat should be complex carbohydrates. Simple carbohydrates simply overwhelm the system.

Fats and oils are a necessary and important part of a healthy diet. Include fats and oils in what you prepare and eat daily but choose wisely. There are healthy and unhealthy oils. **Olive oil** is probably the healthiest oil available for humans. It has more oleic acid (up to 83%), a monounsaturated essential fatty acid (omega 9) than any other oil. Oleic acid is an antioxidant that prevents or slows oxidation both in the bottle and in the body. Oxidation affects the flavor and nutritional value of both our foods and our bodies negatively. Think rancidity. Antioxidants help keep us healthy and fresh.

Oleic acid is the most easily absorbed oil we have, both internally and externally—inside our bodies and also through our skin as an ointment or cream. Remember olive oil is what Christ, the Anointed One, was anointed with. It is good for us inside and out. Olive oil is also beneficial in the treatment of certain illnesses. Oleic acid helps the body fight breast cancer, rheumatoid arthritis, migraine headaches and even type II diabetes. It helps reduce blood pressure and increases the body's fat burning capacity. It is good, good, good. (23)

Oleic acid is also found in avocados, sunflower seeds and peanuts, to name a few good sources. So avocado oil, sunflower oil and peanut oil can also be fairly healthy as long as the oil is cold pressed.

But what about regular old vegetable oils, the kind most people have in their pantries? Don't they also contain nutritious essential fatty acids? No, I'm sorry, they don't. Vegetable oils such as corn oil, soybean oil, safflower, oil, sunflower oil, canola oil and lots of others are processed at high temperatures, not pressed. Heat processing destroys most of the essential fatty acids that occur naturally in unprocessed oils. Only omega 6 fatty acids survive. While omega 6 fatty acids are essential they must be balanced by the omega 3 fatty acids found in fish and a few other foods. Unless the ratio of omega 6 fatty acids to omega 3 fatty acids is in balance omega 6 fatty acids will generate free radicals, negative reactive compounds in the body. These compounds break down lipoproteins, proteins, and DNA. Elevated levels of omega 6 fatty acids cause inflammation and pain. One way to avoid too many omega 6 fatty acids is to avoid all heat-processed oils. (Eliminating processed foods will help too.).

We eat 400 times more omega 6 fatty acids than we did fifty years ago. And we are eating much less fish with its beneficial omega 3 fatty acids. According to the National

Institute of Health, fat and saturated fat intake as a percentage of total calories has decreased for the past three decades while at the same time the intake of omega 6 fatty acids has increased and intake of omega 3 fatty acids has decreased. The ideal ratio of omega 6 to omega 3 fatty acids is 1:1. That ratio today is 20:1 or higher. It is literally sickening. These ratios are all wrong. Most of us are way out of balance. (24)

There are way too many omega-6 fatty acids in the Western diet and too few omega-3 fatty acids. The NIH goes on to point out, "This change in the composition of fatty acids parallels a significant increase in the prevalence of overweight and obesity." (25) This imbalance can also be seen or felt in increased inflammation and pain.

Processed oils are a source of omega 6s. Of course these cheaper oils are used in processed foods and in our own home cooking. We've been told these oils are healthy, but they aren't. Check your pantry. It's time to make a change. You'll feel better when you do!

You may have noticed that I listed sunflower oil as both a healthy and unhealthy oil. What's with that? Oils can be healthy or unhealthy depending on whether they're heat processed or cold-pressed during extraction. Olive oil and a few others are cold- pressed—their oil is physically pressed from the fruit or seed. Avocado oil and grape seed oil are also cold-pressed oils. But almost all other vegetable oils available in the grocery store are heat-processed oils extracted using high temperatures that destroy their nutritional value leaving them dangerously unhealthy. Unfortunately commercial sunflower and peanut oils are usually heat-processed. But both of these oils are sometimes available as cold-pressed oils, usually in specialty stores. Read labels. Shop carefully.

Even olive oil is only cold-pressed in the first two stages—extra virgin and virgin. Then the seeds are heat-processed to remove any remaining oil. The antioxidants and omega 9 fatty acids are destroyed in processing and most of the nutritional value is lost. Only buy and use extra virgin or virgin olive oil. Again, read the labels.

This week shop and cook with healthy oils. I use olive oil in everything from fried eggs to homemade bread. I also cook with butter and coconut oil. Reassess and replace the oils in your cupboard with healthier unprocessed alternatives.

What about, **nuts, seeds, and spices**? These foods are really a part of the fruits, vegetables, roots, and vines we already know are healthy. I only want to mention nuts, seeds and spices as a separate group because they are so incredibly high in antioxidants. Don't ignore these wonderful foods and flavor enhancers. Buy trail mix (check the ingredients!) and keep a jar or a bowl handy for snacking. Add spices to everything. Spices add more than flavor. They are one of the best sources of antioxidants; they help preserve food and keep it fresh and tasty longer.

Then they do that same thing to our insides; they help keep our cells young and fresh. This should be the easiest addition to this week's chart.

One good way to add antioxidants to your diet is with herbal teas. There are many delicious herbal teas available from ginger to turmeric. A cup of lemon ginger or Korean ginseng tea is perfect at bedtime or in the morning. Because some spices found in herbal teas are not absorbed readily without a source of fat, I sometimes add a dollop of cream to my tea, but no sugar.

Finally, with this new healthy eating plan do we need vitamin and mineral **supplements**? I do use a few supplements for several reasons. First, I haven't always eaten the way I do now, hence supplements. Those who once followed or are still eating the typical American diet have a lifetime of nutritional deficiencies. And for those who have spent a lifetime eating in as healthy a way as possible, many fresh fruits, vegetables, meats, and dairy are not as nutritious as they once were. I once read that an orange from 1940 had eight times the nutrients as an orange today. I don't know if that's true. How could it be possible? Different farming techniques, different levels of synthetic fertilizers, different levels of pesticide use, and more. I guess it might be true. Produce, eggs and dairy products, and even fish are mass-produced in conditions that favor the farmer and efficiency but that are not always conducive to nutrition. Dairy products contain antibiotics and hormones. So do beef and chicken, but we've cut back on meat. If you raise chickens for eggs in your backyard you may notice the birds scratch in the dirt, and eat worms and bugs, and there is a difference in the color and flavor of the eggs you gather compared to eggs from the grocery store. Your backyard eggs are more nutritious than the mass-produced eggs most of us buy. So yes, the nutrition available in various foods has and does change.

Supplements are not a solution to maintaining good health; they are what the name says they are, a supplement to a healthy diet. I take fish oil and a probiotic and magnesium every day. I read recently that the microbes in the gut help synthesize some vitamins and that they can benefit from vitamin supplementation. An in depth look at supplements is beyond the scope of this book, but in general I recommend finding a good probiotic for gut health, and fish oil for the brain. There is a huge difference in the quality of what is available. Do some research.

1. Did I have 3 to 4 cups of leafy greens today and at least one serving of fruit?
2. Did I add fish several days this week?
3. Did I eat whole grains for breakfast? Am I only using whole grain breads?
4. Have I added root and vine fruits and vegetables? Did I eat legumes at least once this week?
5. Have I eliminated processed foods?
6. Have I added eggs and lo-fat dairy to enhance my diet?

7. Am I using healthy oils? Is honey my only caloric sweetener? Have I added nuts and spices?

Step 1	M	T	W	Th	F	S	Su
Greens							
Fruit							
Step 2							
Fish							
Step 3							
Breads							
Cereal							
Step 4							
Vines							
Roots							
Legumes							
Step 5							
No process							
Step 6							
Eggs							
Dairy							
Step 7							
Healthy oil							
Honey							
Nuts spice							

Am I ready for Step 8?

16 STEP 8: DRINKS

I saved Step 8, drinks, until nearly last. I have tried to be positive and focus on the wonderful foods we are adding to our diets as we replace less healthy foods. So I will begin by saying DRINK WATER! Positively drink water! Water is what our bodies need. It is a wonderful, miraculous, healthful drink. And besides water, drink milk if you like it. And make flavor infused waters by adding cucumber slices or watermelon chunks or lemon slices. But, and you could see this coming, DON'T drink sugary soft drinks, carbonated drinks, athletic drinks, Gator drinks or Power drinks. Read the ingredient list on any one of these flavored drinks. They are nutrient-free or nearly nutrient-free. They are not good for you, but they do contain lots of sweeteners either with or without calories.

You really could see this coming, couldn't you!

About two hours into a road trip I used to believe without a doubt that I needed a cola drink to continue traveling safely. It took me some time to convince myself it wasn't true. I was finally able to travel without that caffeinated drink by taking water with me everywhere I went. When I thought I needed to stop for a big drink. I drank water. And eventually I saw that I was mostly thirsty and my brain had learned that the answer to thirst on the road came in a 32-ounce cup.

What's wrong with a cold, sugary drink containing no nutrients? It has artificial colors, preservatives, and artificial flavors that water doesn't have. But aside from that, the sugars whether in the form of sucrose or high fructose corn syrup are not good for you. We've already been over this. Other than salt, which our bodies need and which the Israelites had in abundance, sugar is the only legal purely chemical substance humans consume regularly. And we eat a lot of it. Stop! Sugar is intimately associated with both type II diabetes and heart disease as well as with a cluster of other metabolic abnormalities. Eliminating sugar from the diet is one of the best things you can do to improve overall health and well-being. I'm repeating myself here. Stop drinking sugar waters!

Cutting out sugar-sweetened drinks is one of the biggest steps you can take toward improved health. If you follow only this step and no other you will be somewhat healthier. I am not recommending that you take only this step. In fact let me remind you to keep eating greens every day, fish regularly, whole grains, fruits and vegetables. Let me remind you to cook with healthy oils and eliminate processed foods of all kinds. And now on top of that drink water!

Of course you could substitute artificially sweetened drinks for sugary drinks and you might be better off than you are with the sugar, but maybe still not really healthy. No, unfortunately artificial sweeteners carry a lot of baggage of their own. For example artificial sweeteners play havoc with the bacteria in the gut. Recent studies suggest that almost all artificial sweeteners have a negative impact on the intestinal biome. Very recent research suggests that artificial sweeteners can induce glucose intolerance and put you at greater risk for metabolic syndrome and type II diabetes, the very things we are trying to avoid by giving up sugars. In fact artificial sweeteners may be even more likely to induce glucose intolerance than pure sugar. So good-bye Coke Zero. Oh well.

Drink water. Add herbal teas. Add milk instead of sugar. Add fruit. If you drink fruit juices, read the label. Many fruit juices are full of added sugars. Bummer. And even fruit juices without added sugars concentrate the amount of fructose you would normally get from fruit. So, don't have a lot of fruit juice. Have an orange; it's more satisfying.

This week: No carbonated drinks, no sugary drinks. Drink

water morning, noon, and night modified to taste.

1. Did I have 2 to 4 cups of leafy greens today and at least one serving of fruit?
2. Did I add fish several days this week?
3. Did I eat whole grains for breakfast? Am I only using whole grain breads?
4. Have I added root and vine fruits and vegetables? Did I eat legumes this week?
5. Have I eliminated processed foods?
6. Have I added eggs and low fat dairy to enhance my diet?
7. Am I only using healthy oils? Is honey my only caloric sweetener? Have I added nuts, spices?
8. Have I eliminated sugary drinks and added water?

Step 1	M	T	W	Th	F	S	Su
Greens							
Fruit							
Step 2							
Fish							
Step 3							
Breads							
Cereal							
Step 4							

Vines							
Roots							
Legumes							
Step 5							
Nothing							
Step 6							
Eggs							
Dairy							
Step 7							
Healthy oil							
Honey							
Nuts spice							
Step 8							
Water							

Am I ready for Step 9?

17   STEP 9: EXERCISE

*18 And all saints who remember to keep and do these sayings, **walking** in obedience to the commandments, shall receive health in their navel and marrow to their bones;*

19 And shall find wisdom and great treasures of knowledge, even hidden treasures;

20 And shall run and not be weary, and shall walk and not faint.

21And I, the Lord, give unto them a promise, that the destroying angel shall pass by them, as the children of Israel, and not slay them. Amen.

There are many benefits to exercise. Exercise plays an important role in regulating blood sugar and improving the ability of receptor cells to utilize insulin. Exercise helps build bone density and thus overcome bone loss in osteoporosis. Exercise affects the ratio of **H**DL or High Density Lipoproteins (think **H**ealthy DL) to **L**DL or Low Density Lipoproteins (think **L**ousy DL) and may help to maintain a healthy HDL to LDL ratio. It may require more exercise than walking from the car to the living room, and even more exercise than pushing the vacuum around the house or yelling at Alexa to change the channel to reap the benefits. But a nice walk four or five days a week will definitely help and it can be a social activity.

Exercise builds muscles. No surprise there. We lose muscle naturally as we age. You wondered why it's harder to move the furniture around? Aging also increases the risk of developing type II diabetes for a number of reasons. But consider this: muscle tissue acts as a reservoir for the glucose the body draws on to keep blood glucose levels stable. Less muscle means less glucose storage, and greater difficulty in regulating blood glucose levels. This is just one reason exercise is so directly important in overall health and in avoiding type II diabetes specifically.

Exercise is beneficial in combatting many diseases, from a reduced risk of cancer to a sense of overall mental and physical well-being. Exercise helps reduce stress and clears the mind. Exercise may raise your spirits along with your energy levels. Exercise brings increased oxygen to the muscles and increases the size and number of our mitochondria—the energy producers in our cells. Exercise, rather than sapping energy, helps us become more energetic.

Even a moderate amount of exercise can measurably increase longevity. My great grandmother walked across the plains to Salt Lake City. She raised twelve children and lived to be 104. Was exercise one of the factors in her long life? Exercise may not make us centenarians, but it can make life better.

What type of exercise should you be doing? Do what works for you. If you love yoga and tai chi join a group. But generally brisk walking provides all the benefits of exercise. My only suggestion comes from an energetic walker: "Start your exercise program the way a little child plays. Kids don't do the same thing for too long. They run, walk, stop, turn, skip and jump. Just move. Walk and run and if something hurts stop doing it for a while." I think this is good advice whether you're walking, running, swimming, playing tennis, or riding a horse. Whatever you're doing, try to enjoy yourself. I remember many years ago walking to church with my little sister. We hadn't gone very far when she turned to me and said in a whiny voice, "I'm tired of walking." Then she brightened up as an idea came to her: "Let's run a while," and off she went.

1. Did I have 2 to 4 cups of leafy greens today and at least one serving of fruit?
2. Did I add fish several days this week?

3. Did I eat whole grains for breakfast? Am I only using whole grain breads?

4. Have I added root and vine fruits and vegetables? Did I eat legumes at least once this week?

5. Have I eliminated processed foods?

6. Have I added eggs and lo-fat dairy to enhance my diet?

7. Am I only using healthy oils? Is honey my only caloric sweetener? Have I added nuts and spices?

8. Have I eliminated sugary drinks and added water?

9. Am I moving, walking or running?

Step 1	M	T	W	Th	F	S	Su
Greens							
Fruit							
Step 2							
Fish							
Step 3							
Breads							
Cereal							
Step 4							
Vines							
Roots							
Legumes							
Step 5							
No process							

Step 6							
Eggs							
Dairy							
Step 7							
Healthy oil							
Honey							
Nuts spice							
Step 8							
Water							
Step 9							
Exercise							

18 REVIEW

This isn't really a chapter. This is just a reminder and a way to put this all together. You are beginning to understand the Word of Wisdom in a whole new way. You have set goals and taken steps to follow a new way of eating. Maybe you don't agree with me on everything. That's fine. Make this a program you can follow, and don't stop now. Keep motivated! Go back and remind yourself of what it is you're doing and why. Look better, feel better, and follow the commandments.

Remember: drink plenty of water and avoid sweetened soft drinks, sodas and fruit juice. Enjoy healthy fats and don't skip the salt. You're not getting nearly as much salt as you did when you ate processed foods! If you feel hungry, eat healthy snacks between meals. If you wait to eat until you're really hungry it's harder to stick to the plan and easier to turn to less healthy snacks. When you cut back on processed foods you will be cutting back on sugar and white flour automatically, and vice versa!

Eat three or four cups of green leafy vegetables every day. Enjoy vegetable juices like tomato juice and V-8. Enjoy fresh fruits, starchy vegetables, legumes and whole grains. Enhance your food with milk, cheese, butter and yogurt. Eat eggs, nuts, seeds and fish. Use coconut and olive oils. Eat your fruits and vegetables fresh or frozen. Add spices. Spices are full of antioxidants and full of flavor.

Just a final note: In the preceding chapters I assume you eat three meals a day. But there are other eating schedules you may choose to follow. A three meal a day plan with two snacks can easily become a five meal a day plan. It shouldn't make much difference unless you suffer from high blood sugar, in which case five small meals may help regulate blood sugar better than three larger, more traditional meals.

Scholars believe that at the time of Christ folks generally ate only two meals a day—midmorning and late afternoon. I'm sometimes on that schedule if I sleep in! But generally I think it matters more what you eat throughout the day than how many meals you divide it into. At the end of the book following the recipes is a full page chart if you want to copy it off and keep it on your fridge. In the meantime, whatever else you do, enjoy!

1. Did I have 2 to 3 cups of leafy greens today and 2 or more servings of fruit?
2. Did I add fish several days this week?

3. Did I eat whole grains for breakfast? Am I only using whole grain breads?
4. Have I added root and vine fruits and vegetables? Did I eat legumes at least once this week?
5. Have I eliminated processed foods?
6. Have I added eggs and dairy to enhance my diet?
7. Am I only using healthy oils? Is honey my only caloric sweetener? Have I added nuts and spices?
8. Have I eliminated sugary drinks and added water?
9. Am I moving, walking or running?

THIS WEEK DO IT ALL AGAIN!

Step 1	M	T	W	Th	F	S	Su
Greens							
Fruit							
Step 2							
Fish							
Step 3							
Breads							
Cereal							
Step 4							
Vines							
Roots							
Legumes							

Step 5							
No process							
Step 6							
Eggs							
Dairy							
Step 7							
Healthy oil							
Honey							
Nuts spice							
Step 8							
Water							
Step 9							
Exercise							

Make the Breakthrough

Stay above the line!

Fresh fruits and vegetables

Roots, grains and legumes

Fish and eggs

Dairy: milk and butter

Cheese and yogurt

Olive oil

_____

Meat

Sugary drinks

All refined sugars

Highly processed foods

Refined grains and white flour

Processed vegetable oils

19 SAMPLE MEALS AND MORE

Here you'll find some helpful tips, meal guides and other useful information.

Let's start with <u>wholesome herbs</u>: (Remember to eat 2 to 4 cups every day)
This is not a comprehensive list by any means. But all of these wholesome herbs are chock full of nutrients and have been shown to be microbiome and mycobiome friendly. (They help both good bacteria and good fungi to flourish in the gut.) Eat these every day. And add to this list as much as you want.

Artichokes	Cucumber
Asparagus	Dandelion Greens
Beet Greens	Egg Plant
Celery	Endive
Chicory	Garlic

Cilantro

Lettuces, all types

Mushrooms

Onions, leeks, chives

Parsley

Parsnips

Peppers

Purslane

Grape Leaves

Radicchio

Shallots

Sorrel

Spinach

Squash Blossoms

Swiss Chard

Tomatoes

Cruciferous vegetables are wholesome herbs that deserve a category of their own. Cruciferous vegetables are by definition members of the cabbage family. These plants are so beneficial to us health wise it would be a good idea to add them to every meal in addition to the plants in the list above. Plan to eat at least a cup or more of cruciferous vegetables as a part of your daily diet:

Arugula

Broccoli

Cabbages, all types

Collard Greens

Kale

Mustard Greens

Rutabaga

Turnip Greens

Bok Choy

Brussels Sprouts

Cauliflower

Jicama

Kohlrabi

Radishes, all types

Turnips

Watercress

    And many others.

Next we need to consider *whole grains, and the "fruit of the vine whether in the ground or above the ground"*. Many grains, roots and vine plants contain a special kind of carbohydrate known as <u>resistant starch</u>. This resistant starch is not digested in the stomach or in the small intestine. It travels all the way to the large intestine where it is broken down by and feeds the healthy microbes that help our bodily systems to grow and function properly, including the immune system. I recommend eating resistant starches at every meal. It could be the oatmeal for your breakfast, or the whole wheat toast with your scrambled eggs. It might be the refried beans in your corn tortilla—oh, corn is a resistant starch too! It is easy to add these foods every time you eat:

Unripe Bananas	Corn, whole grain
Legumes, all types	Oats
Potatoes	Rice, brown
Soy products	Sweet potatoes
Winter squashes	Yams

Whole grains and 100% whole grain Multi grain products including:

Sprouted grains	Barley
Millet	Quinoa
Rye	Wheat

Berries and other fruits that fall into the vine category do not provide resistant starches. But berries are an excellent source of phytonutrients and should also be a part of your regular diet.

Sample Meals:

I try to have all the essential nutrients with every meal, that is proteins, fats, carbohydrates, fiber, and water. These sample menus are designed with that in mind.

BREAKFAST

I.   2 eggs scrambled with ½ cup spinach, ½ cup mushrooms, ¼ cup onions, and then sprinkled with a handful of grated cheese. Add ½ cup refried beans or 1 slice whole wheat toast. 1 cup herbal tea and 1 piece of fruit.

II. ½ cup old-fashioned oats cooked in 1 cup water with ½ cup low fat milk. Add 1 cup blueberries. 1 hard cooked egg or 2 eggs scrambled or fried in olive oil. Herbal tea.

III. Berry smoothie made with low fat milk or almond milk, 2 cups berries, juice from ½ a lemon, 1 handful of chopped kale or spinach, ½ cup ice and water as needed. One slice whole wheat toast.

LUNCH

I.   Big salad with wholesome herbs of your choice, protein from fish, beans, or tofu, Sprinkle with cheese or nuts or seeds as a topping. Add olive oil salad dressing to taste. One slice whole wheat bread. Herbal tea or sparkling water.

II.   Big salad as above. Black bean soup. I piece of fruit. Herbal teas or sparkling water.

III.   Tuna salad sandwich on whole wheat bread. Mix tuna with chopped celery and walnuts. Spread between lettuce slices on bread. Chilean onion and tomato salad on side. Sparkling water.

DINNER

I.   6 oz. grilled salmon over brown rice, steamed asparagus, steamed broccoli. Soup.

II.   Fish tacos on corn tortillas. Serve with coleslaw made from 1 cup chopped cabbage; I grated carrot, 1 minced green onion, 1 minced garlic clove and ½ cup low fat yogurt. Add fresh tomato based salsa and refried beans.

III.   Minestrone soup topped with Parmesan cheese with 1 slice whole wheat bread. Herbal tea.

SNACKS

If you feel hungry during the day snack on raw veggies—carrot sticks, celery sticks with peanut butter, broccoli florets, hummus, leftover salads or soups, plain yogurt, nuts or grapes or berries, cheese sticks, and so on. Try to include protein and fat with each snack. There are lots of healthy foods you can snack on. And of course you can add any of these snacks to any of your meals.

To help in meal planning it might be good to have a list of protein and fat sources as well as the wholesome herbs and other fruits and vegetables already listed. These are pretty good lists but they are not comprehensive. Feel free to add to them foods that fit the bill for good health and nutrition.

Protein

(Have at least 3 servings daily, 4 if you have a snack)

Eggs	Fish
Shellfish	Cheese, low fat
Cottage Cheese	Yogurts, Plain low fat
Soy products	Peanuts
Legumes	Other nuts and seeds

Fats(Have at least 3 servings daily, 4 if you have a snack)

Avocado oil

Coconut oil

Olive oil, extra virgin

Flaxseed oil

Ghee

Grapeseed oil

Hemp oil

Nut oils

Nut butters

Safflower oil

Sesame oil

Coconut milk, canned

Eggs

Fatty fish

Nuts

Tofu

All oils should be cold pressed, not heat processes. This eliminates many of the vegetable oils you may have been using.

Another good way to keep track of what you eat now that you are eating the Lord's way is to track the nutrients you have at every meal. Every meal should include protein, fat, carbohydrates, fiber and water. (Our bodies can only digest so much protein at any one time. It has to be added regularly. The same is true for all the essential nutrients.)

Carbohydrates should include wholesome herbs and resistant starches, or in other words, grains, roots, and the fruits of the vine. If you are eating these complex carbs you will have the fiber you need. If you drink water with every meal either plain or with an herbal tea, your body will have the hydration it needs. Snacks should at the very least have a protein and a fat source.

MEALS	Mon	Tues	Wed	Thurs	Fri	Sat	Sun
Breakfast							
Protein							
Fat							
Vines Roots							
Wholesome herbs							
Water							
Lunch							
Protein							
Fat							
Vines Roots							
Wholesome Herbs							
Water							
Dinner							
Protein							
Fat							
Vines Roots							
Wholesome Herbs							
Water							
Snacks							
Protein							
Fat							
Water							

20 WHAT IS KOSHER?

Kosher or Kashrut is a set of biblical dietary rules or restrictions governing both food preparation and consumption. The word Kashrut comes from the Hebrew letters Kaf-Shin-Riesh and means *fit and proper* or *correct*. Kosher then refers to the correct and proper way to prepare and eat food, and specifies foods that meet this standard. The word kosher can also to be used to describe objects that are correctly made in accordance with law and are therefore fit for ritual use. I will mention here only the kosher laws from the Bible, but will not comment on the expanded interpretations from the Talmud.

Food is not blessed by a rabbi to make it kosher. It is either kosher by definition and preparation or it is not. The vegetables in your garden are kosher as long as you don't have bugs! Bugs aren't kosher. Kosher laws are observed year round at every meal and with every bite of food. Passover has additional kosher laws that pertain specifically to the Passover week. For example, only unleavened bread is acceptable during Passover. Unleavened bread is kosher all year, and leavened bread is kosher except during Passover. Many of the kosher restrictions are beneficial in terms of better health and sanitation. But not all. Like the Word of Wisdom, kosher rules are followed because they come from God, not because science has shown them to be the healthiest or best practices in every case. We show our obedience to God by following the laws he has given us in and for our time.

Rabbi Hayim Halevy Donin, in his book *To Be a Jew (24)* explains that the dietary laws are given as a call to holiness. Our ability to distinguish between right and wrong, good and evil, pure and defiled, the sacred and the profane is very important in religion. According to Donin imposing rules on what you can and cannot eat requires a person to control even the most basic and primal instincts.

Perhaps the same could be said for the Word of Wisdom, which though specifically given as a guide to good health requires a degree of obedience and control.

The kosher laws as given in scripture are fairly straightforward. Leviticus, Numbers, and Deuteronomy all contain these laws and repeat the same basic information. The firsts seven chapters of Leviticus, the Book of Laws, set out the regulations governing animal sacrifice. Then in chapter eight Aaron and his sons are washed and anointed and consecrated to officiate in the temple. In chapter nine they offer sacrifices for all of Israel and in chapter ten two men offer unauthorized sacrifices and are struck dead. Also in chapter ten Aaron and his sons are commanded to abstain from wine and other strong drinks. Finally in chapter eleven the Lord reveals which living things may and may not be eaten. Certain animals are classified as clean while others are classified as unclean.

> *Whatsoever parteth the hoof, and is cloven footed, and cheweth the cud, among the beasts, that shall ye eat.*

Cattle, sheep, goats, deer, and bison both chew their cud and have a cloven hoof; they are kosher and can be eaten. In Leviticus 11: 4-8, the Lord specifies certain animals which are not kosher so that there can be no mistakes or rationalizations:

> *Nevertheless these shall ye not eat of them that chew the cud, or of them that divide the hoof: as the camel, because he cheweth the cud, but divideth not the hoof; he is unclean unto you.*

> *And the coney, (rabbit) because he cheweth the cud, but divideth not the hoof; he is unclean unto you. And the hare, because he cheweth the cud, but divideth not the hoof; he is unclean unto you. And the swine (there goes pork), though he divide the hoof, and be cloven footed, yet he cheweth not the cud; he is unclean to you. Of their flesh shall ye not*

eat, and their carcasses shall ye not touch; they are unclean to you.

The camel, rabbit, hare and pig were specified as unclean, not to be eaten or even touched.

Leviticus 7: 23-27 specifies that even with acceptable animals, the fat and blood should not be eaten, nor should animals that have died of natural or unnatural causes other than ritual slaughter be eaten.

We are not governed by these laws today; nobody will be disfellowshipped for eating blood or animal fat, but it is interesting to note what was and was not allowable.

Leviticus 11: 9-12 regulates fish and shellfish:

> *These shall ye eat of all that are in the waters: whatsoever hath fins and scales in the waters, in the seas, and in the rivers, them shall ye eat. And all that have not fins and scales in the seas, and in the rivers, of all that move in the waters, and of any living thing which is in the waters, they shall be an abomination unto you: They shall be even an abomination unto you; ye shall not eat of their flesh, but ye shall have their carcasses in abomination. Whatsoever hath no fins nor scales in the waters, that shall be an abomination unto you.*

So fish with scales are good whether from the sea or from

the river. But shellfish such as lobster, oysters, shrimp, clams, and crabs are not kosher. Neither are fish without fins or scales. Sharks and eels and so on are not kosher. Fish, unlike beasts and fowls, do not have to be ritually slaughtered and their fat and blood are acceptable and can be eaten. Fish are good as long as they have fins and scales.

Leviticus 11: 13-19 specifies a number of birds that are not acceptable:

> *And these are they which ye shall have in abomination among the fowls; they shall not be eaten, they are an abomination: the eagle, and the ossifrage, and the ospray, And the vulture, and the kite after his kind; Every raven after his kind; And the owl, and the night hawk, and the cuckow, and the hawk after his kind, And the little owl, and the cormorant, and the great owl, And the swan, and the pelican, and the gier eagle, And the stork, the heron after her kind, and the lapwing, and the bat.*

All the birds listed are birds of prey or scavengers and so it has been inferred that this was the basis for the distinction. Other birds were permitted including chickens, geese, ducks, and turkeys. This is clarified in Deuteronomy 14: 20 which simply says, *But of all clean fowls ye may eat.*

Reptiles, rodents, amphibians, and insects (winged

swarming things) are all forbidden in Leviticus 11: 20-30, with the exception of a few insects listed in Leviticus 11: 22:

> *Even these of them ye may eat; the locust after his kind, and the bald locust after his kind, and the beetle after his kind, and the grasshopper after his kind.*

So no more rattlesnake steaks, but grasshoppers are fine. No part of a forbidden animal may be eaten. Any product derived from forbidden animals such as milk, eggs, fat, or organs is also forbidden.

Verses 31-38 explain cleanliness rules for the pots, pans, stove and water that may come in contact with unclean creatures or conditions. For example verse 33 explains that any earthen vessel that falls to the ground becomes unclean and must be broken. You've got to be careful in the kitchen! Verse 39 restates the prohibition against eating animals that have died rather than being slaughtered. No road kill! This is clarified again in Deuteronomy 14: 21:

> *Ye shall not eat of any thing that dieth of itself: thou shalt give it unto the stranger that is in thy gates that he may eat it; or thou mayest sell it unto an alien: for thou art an holy people unto the Lord thy God. Thou shalt not seethe a kid in his mother's milk.*

Oh, and by the way, don't boil a young goat in its mother's milk. This admonition is repeated three times in the Old Testament. Rabbinical law has interpreted this to mean milk and meat should never be eaten together (excluding fish), although that distinction is not made in the Old Testament itself. Finally, all fruits and vegetables are kosher.

Leviticus 11: 44-47 explains that these regulations are given by God to make his people holy, and certainly the same could be said for the Word of Wisdom :

> *For I am the Lord your God: ye shall therefore sanctify yourselves, and ye shall be holy; for I am holy: neither shall ye defile yourselves with any manner of creeping thing that creepeth upon the earth. For I am the Lord that bringeth you up out of the land of Egypt, to be your God: ye shall therefore be holy, for I am holy. This is the law of the beasts, and of the fowl, and of every living creature that moveth in the waters, and of every creature that creepeth upon the earth: To make a difference between the unclean and the clean, and between the beast that may be eaten and the beast that may not be eaten.*

21 RECIPES

Some helpful hints: When I use whole wheat flour in baked goods I always buy white wheat whole wheat flour, not red. White wheat makes lighter breads and cakes, etc. White wheat may be the source of the fine flour mentioned in the Bible.

I use white flour to thicken sauces or gravies. I think of white flour as a non-nutritive filler. If you want nutrition go with whole grain flours.

When I specify buttermilk in a recipe it is usually interchangeable with yogurt. Both are acidic, which is what the recipe is asking for. As a matter of convenience I often use low fat yogurt because that's what I have on hand

We live in a really easy time for cooks. We can buy grated cheese, grated carrots and broccoli, chopped greens and prepackaged salads. I use an instant pot and a bread maker. But any of these recipes can be made with or without fancy machines and simplified store prep and packaging. Do what works for you.

A number of these recipes use honey. I try to minimize the use of honey because I really think it has to be used sparingly. It is a sweet treat, not an everyday addition.

Don't buy foods you don't want to eat. Don't even bring foods into the house if they don't fit your new way of eating. Don't have desserts every day, but enjoy them when you do. The recipes here are fairly healthy.

These recipes are based on a three-meal-a-day eating plan. You can devise a two-meal plan or a five or six-meal-a-day plan if it suits you better. For me it doesn't make much difference how many meals a day I eat as long as I eat nutritious foods. The only disclaimer I'll make here is that if you suffer from elevated blood sugar, five or six small meals a day may keep your blood sugar and insulin under better control than a two or three meal a day plan. More small meals may also help you curb your appetite initially. Do what works for you. And eat before you get really hungry!

BREADS

Apple Muffins

Stir together

> 1 cup whole wheat flour
>
> 1 cup rolled oats
>
> 1/2 tsp salt
>
> 1 tsp baking powder
>
> 1/2 tsp baking soda

Combine and add to dry ingredients

> 2 eggs
>
> 1 tsp vanilla
>
> 1/2 cup honey
>
> 1/4 cup coconut oil
>
> 3/4 cup milk
>
> 1 apple, chopped

Bake in greased muffin cups at 400° for 20 minutes.

Apple Oat Bran Muffins

Stir together

> 1-1/4 cups whole wheat flour
>
> 1 cup oat bran
>
> 2-1/2 tsp baking powder
>
> 1/4 tsp baking soda
>
> 1/4 tsp salt
>
> 1/4 tsp nutmeg
>
> 1/4 tsp cinnamon

Combine and add to dry ingredients

1 cup buttermilk or yogurt

2 eggs

1/4 cup honey

2 Tbsp coconut oil

Stir together just until moistened. Add 3/4 cup apple, peeled and shredded. Bake in greased muffin cups at 375° for 18-20 minutes.

Banana Nut Muffins

Combine in large bowl

1-1/2 cups whole wheat flour

1/2 cup wheat germ

1 cup chopped walnuts

1 Tbsp baking powder

1/2 tsp salt

1 tsp cinnamon

1/4 tsp nutmeg

Stir in, mixing until just blended

2 ripe bananas, mashed

3/4 cup milk

5 Tbsp melted butter

Bake in muffin tins at 400°, 20 to 22 minutes.

Carrot Muffins

In large bowl stir together

      1-1/2 cups whole wheat flour

      2 tsp baking powder

      1/2 tsp salt

In separate bowl beat together

      2 eggs

      2/3 cup yogurt

      1/4 cup honey

      2 Tbsp coconut oil

Stir in 1/2 cup carrots, shredded

Spoon batter into 12 greased muffin cups. Bake at 375° for 15 to 20 minutes.

Cranberry Nut Muffins

Beat 2 eggs

Add   1/2 cup coconut oil

      1/2 cup honey

      1 tsp vanilla

Add   1-1/4 cups whole wheat flour

      1/4 cup oat flour

      1-1/2 tsp baking powder

Do not over mix. Fold in

      3/4 cup dried cranberries

      1/2 cup walnuts, chopped

Pour into 12 muffin cups. Bake at 350° for 25 minutes.

Meem's Banana Bread

Combine in mixing bowl

　　　1 tsp vanilla

　　　3 ripe bananas

Combine and add

　　　1-3⁄4 cups whole wheat flour

　　　1 tsp baking soda

　　　1⁄2 tsp salt

　　　1⁄4 tsp baking powder

While blending on low speed pour in 1 cup evaporated milk.

Blend well on medium

Add　　1⁄2 cup walnuts, chopped

Pour into greased bunt pan, bake at 350° for I hour and fifteen minutes.

Pumpkin Bread

Mix together

　　　3 eggs

　　　2/3 cup honey

　　　1 16 oz can or 2 cups cooked pumpkin

　　　2 cups coconut oil

Combine and add to liquid ingredients

　　　3 cups whole wheat flour

　　　1-1⁄2 tsp cinnamon

　　　1-1⁄2 tsp baking powder

　　　1 tsp baking soda

　　　1 tsp salt

3/4 tsp nutmeg

3/4 tsp cloves

Add   1 cup raisins (optional)

Spoon batter into 2 greased bread pans, bake at 350° for 1 hour and 15 minutes.

Hearty Whole Wheat Bread

Combine in bread maker

1-1/4 cups warm water

1/4 cup butter

1 Tbsp to 1/4 cup honey

Add   2 1/2 cups whole wheat flour

1 rounded Tbsp dough conditioner

1 tsp salt

1/2 cup dry milk (optional)

1 tsp instant yeast

Bake according to machine settings.

Raisin-filled Honey Loaf

Combine

       2 Tbsp active dry yeast

       1-1/2 tsp salt

       1 tsp cinnamon

       2 cup whole wheat flour

Add to dry ingredients

       1-1/4 cups warm milk

       1/4 cup warm water

       1/4 cup honey

       1/4 cup butter

Add   1 egg

       2 cups rolled oats or granola

Knead until smooth and elastic. Cover in oiled bowl. Set aside for 1 1/2 to 2 hours and in the meantime prepare the raisin filling and honey glaze.

Raisin filling:

In saucepan combine

       1 tsp cornstarch

       3 Tbsp honey

Add   I cup raisins, coarsely chopped

       1/2 cup orange juice

       1/2 tsp grated lemon rind

Bring to boil, stir until thickened. Cool

Honey glaze:
Blend 1 Tbsp butter
      1 Tbsp honey

Punch dough down and divide in two. Roll each half into a 9 x 12 inch rectangle. Spread with half the raisin filling. Rollup from the 9-inch end and place in greased loaf pans. Let rise 45 minutes to 1 hour. Bake at 350° for 30 minutes. Spread with honey glaze while warm. Return to oven and bake an additional 10 minutes.

Zucchini-Carrot Bread

Combine and beat together until thick and fluffy
      2 eggs
      1/2 cup coconut oil
      1/4 cup honey
      1-1/2 tsp maple syrup

Stir in with a spoon
      1/2 cup zucchini, shredded
      1/2 cup carrots, shredded

In a separate bowl stir together and fold into zucchini mixture
      1-1/4 cups whole wheat flour
      1/4 cup wheat germ
      1 tsp baking soda
      1 tsp salt
      1/4 tsp baking powder
      1/2 cup chopped walnuts

Pour into greased loaf pan. Sprinkle with 3 Tbsp sesame seeds. Bake at 350° for 1 hour.

BREAKFAST

Breakfast Bake

Sauté 1⁄2 c mushrooms, chopped

      1⁄4 c bell pepper, chopped

      3⁄4 c zucchini, diced

Combine and pour over vegetables:

      6 large eggs

      1 T basil

      1/3 c Parmesan cheese

      salsa to taste

      1 T olive oil

Cook about a minute, then add

      1⁄4 c green onions, diced

      Salt and pepper

Bake in oven at 350° for 7-8 minutes

Breakfast Burrito

Scramble 4 eggs

Toast   3 tortillas in a pan or on the burner

Divide eggs between tortillas

Add shredded cheese and salsa

Wrap and enjoy!

Breakfast Tostada

Divide ingredients between 6 or 7 warm corn tortillas:

      1-1/2 cup shredded lettuce or cabbage

      1 cup diced tomato

      1 large avocado, sliced

      1 1/2 cups cooked beans

Add one fried egg on top of each tostada.

Sprinkle with Shredded cheese, chopped cilantro, and salsa

Fried Eggs with Refried Beans

Fry in medium frying pan 2 eggs

Lower heat and add 3/4 c cooked pinto beans

Top with salsa, cheese and grated cabbage

Karen's Good Granola

Mix together in a large bowl

One 42 ounce drum old-fashioned rolled oats

1 cup wheat germ

1 cup oat bran

1 cup wheat bran

2 cups unsweetened shredded coconut

1/2 cup poppy seeds

1/2 cup sesame seeds

1 cup sunflower seeds

1 cup chopped walnuts

1 cup dry powdered milk

2 Tbsp cinnamon

Combine and heat until liquid

1-1/2 cups coconut oil

2/3 cup honey

1-1/2 tsp salt

1/4 cup water

1 Tbsp vanilla

Pour liquid over dry ingredients. Toss, mixing well. Spread mixture in shallow pans. Bake for 30 minutes at 300°, stirring every ten minutes. Cool and stir in 2 cups of raisins or other dried fruit.

.

Yummy Whole Grain Pancake Mix

(This is a make-ahead mix and will make enough for several meals.)

Combine in mixing bowl

  5 cups whole wheat flour

  3 cups old fashioned rolled oats (chopped, but not powdered, in food processor)

  3 Tbsp baking powder

  1 Tbsp salt

  1 Tbsp baking soda

Warm to combine honey and oil

  1 cup coconut oil

  2 Tbsp honey

Turning bowl as you work, drizzle oil/honey mixture over dry ingredients and cut in. Store in an airtight container in the refrigerator.

Yummy Whole-Grain Pancakes

Whisk together

  1 cup Yummy Whole Grain Pancake Mix

  1 cup buttermilk **OR**

  1/2 cup yogurt and 1/2 cup milk

  1 egg

Let stand for 10 to 15 minutes as batter thickens. Heat griddle to 350° or on medium hot. Drop batter in 1/4 cupsful. When bubbles form on the surface (about 2 minutes) turn the pancakes and cook on the second side (also about 2 minutes). Serve immediately!

DESSERTS, SNACKS

Apple Pandowdy

Peel, slice and arrange in greased, shallow baking dish

> 4 cups tart apples (4 to 5 apples)

In saucepan combine and stir over low heat

> 1/2 cup honey
>
> 1/4 cup flour
>
> 1 tsp cinnamon
>
> 1/4 tsp nutmeg
>
> 1/4 tsp salt
>
> 3/4 cup water

Add   2 Tbsp butter

> 1 Tbsp lemon juice

Pour sauce over sliced apples.

Dough:

Mix together

> 1 cup whole wheat flour
>
> 1/2 tsp salt
>
> 2 tsp baking powder

Cut in

> 4 Tbsp butter

Add   about 2/3 cup yogurt

> (enough liquid to make a soft dough)

Spoon dough over apples making 8 biscuits. Bake at 350° for 40 minutes or until biscuits are browned and apples are tender. Serve warm.

Apple Pudding Cake

Combine ingredients in medium bowl

    2 cups chopped apples (2 or 3 apples)

    1/2 cup honey

    1/4 cup melted butter

Let apples stand for 1 hour then add

    1 cup whole wheat flour

    1 tsp baking soda

    1/2 tsp cinnamon

    1/2 tsp nutmeg

    I egg, beaten and stirred into batter

Bake in an 8 x 8 inch pan at 350° for 35 minutes.

Applesauce Cake

Combine in large bowl

    1/2 cup butter

    1/2 cup honey

    1 tsp vanilla

Combine dry ingredients and add alternately with applesauce

    1 cup unsweetened applesauce

    2 cups whole wheat flour

    1 tsp baking soda

    1/2 tsp nutmeg

    1 tsp cinnamon

    1/2 tsp ground cloves

    3/4 cup dates, chopped

    1 cup walnuts, chopped

Bake at 350°

Blueberry Cake

Whisk together in medium bowl

> 1/2 cup yogurt
>
> 3 eggs
>
> 1 tsp lemon zest
>
> 1 tsp vanilla

Add honey and oil and stir until smooth

> 2/3 cup honey
>
> 1/2 cup coconut oil

Combine dry ingredients and stir in

> 1-1/2 cups whole wheat flour
>
> 2 tsp baking powder
>
> 1/2 tsp salt

Fold in 2 cups fresh or frozen blueberries.

Bake at 350° for 70 to 75 minutes.

Large Chocolate Cake

Combine

> 1 cup coconut oil
>
> 2/3 cup honey
>
> 2 eggs

Add, and mix in on low speed

> 2-1/2 cups whole wheat flour
>
> 2 tsp baking soda
>
> 1/2 tsp salt
>
> 1/2 cup baking cocoa powder

Beat in 1 cup boiling water

Pour into pan, bake at 350° for 35 minutes. Delicious!

Oatmeal Cookies

Cream together

       1-1/3 cups honey

       3⁄4 cup butter

       1⁄4 cup coconut oil

Add and stir in

       2 tsp vanilla

       3 Tbsp milk

       2-1⁄2 cups old fashioned oats

       2-1⁄2 cups whole wheat flour

       1 tsp baking soda

       1 tsp baking powder

       1 tsp salt

Add (optional)

       2 cups cranberries or raisins

       1 cup coconut shredded

       1 cup nuts, chopped

Bake at 375° for 12 to 15 minutes. Cool on cookie sheet

Poppy Seed Cake

Mix together in large bowl

       1 cup honey

       3⁄4 cup coconut oil

       3 eggs

       1 tsp vanilla

Combine dry ingredients alternating with milk

       1 cup milk

       3 cups whole wheat flour

       1 1⁄2 tsp soda

Combine wet and dry ingredients

Add   1⁄2 cup poppy seeds

       1 cup chopped walnuts

Bake in well-greased tube pan at 350° for 1 hour and 15 minutes.

Spicy Whole Wheat Bars

Combine

       1⁄2 cup honey

       1/3 cup coconut oil

       1 egg

In separate bowl combine

       1 cup whole wheat flour

       1⁄4 cup wheat germ

       1⁄2 tsp baking soda

       1⁄2 tsp cinnamon

       1⁄4 tsp cloves

       1⁄4 tsp salt

Combine wet and dry ingredients. Stir in

       1⁄2 cup yogurt or buttermilk

Add   1⁄2 cup dates or raisins, chopped

       1⁄2 cup walnuts, chopped

Pour into greased 9 inch square pan. Bake at 350° for 35 to 40 minutes.

Banana Popsicles

Blend together, mold and freeze 2 bananas

1⁄4 cup yogurt 1⁄4 cup milk

Savory Pecans

Preheat oven to 350°. In a small bowl combine

> 1/2 tsp salt
>
> 1/2 tsp black pepper
>
> 1/2 tsp red pepper flakes
>
> 1/2 tsp chili powder
>
> 1/4 tsp cumin

In a medium skillet over medium heat, melt

> 6 Tbsp butter

Add   2 cups pecan halves

Toss and coat, then toss in combined spices. Spread on cookie sheet and bake for 45 minutes. Set oven to broil and crisp nuts for 3 to 5 minutes. Use to top vegetable and other dishes, or eat as a snack.

Toasted Pumpkin Seeds

Mix all ingredients in a bowl

> 2 cups clean dry pumpkins seeds
>
> 1-1/2 tsp olive oil
>
> 1 1/2 tsp salt

Spread coated seeds on cookie sheet. Bake at 250° until crispy stirring occasionally.

DRINKS

Apple Smoothie

Combine

> 1 cup milk or yogurt
>
> 2 apples, chopped
>
> 2 cups greens
>
> 2/3 cup parsley
>
> 1/3 cup cilantro
>
> 1/2 avocado
>
> 2 tsp lemon juice
>
> 1 cup ice cubes Blend until smooth

Avocado Smoothie

Combine

> 1 cup milk or yogurt
>
> 1/2 avocado
>
> 1 ripe banana
>
> 1 Tbsp chia seeds
>
> 1/2 tsp cinnamon
>
> 1/4 tsp vanilla
>
> 1 scoop protein powder (optional)
>
> 1 heaping tsp psyllium (optional)

Blend together with 1 cup ice cubes

Serve and enjoy.

Fruit Nog

Combine in blender

1 ripe banana or1 peach, or other fruit, peeled

1 egg

3 Tbsp wheat germ or 1 Tbsp psyllium

1/2 tsp vanilla

Blend together until ingredients are smooth.

Berry Smoothie

Combine

>2 cups frozen berries
>
>1 cup yogurt
>
>1/2 cup milk
>
>1/2 cup orange juice
>
>1 tsp vanilla

Blend until smooth.

Almond Raspberry Smoothie

Combine

>1/2 cup plain full fat yogurt
>
>1/2 cup raspberries
>
>1/4 cup slivered almonds
>
>1/2 cup milk

Puree until smooth and creamy.

Blueberry smoothie

Combine

      1 cup plain low-fat yogurt

      1⁄2 cup frozen blueberries

      2 Tbsp black cherry juice

      1⁄2 Tbsp plain psyllium

Puree until smooth and creamy.

Carbonated Drinks

Fill a cup with ice and club soda Add 100% fruit juice to taste

EGGS

Artichoke Frittata

Heat oven to 400°.

Heat in frying pan over medium heat

    2 Tbsp olive oil

Whisk together and add

    8 eggs

    2 cloves garlic, chopped

    1/2 cup plain yogurt

    salt and pepper

Add 1 cup Parmesan cheese

    2 Tbsp fresh rosemary

    12 oz artichoke hearts, drained

Cook on stove top for 3 to 4 minutes. Transfer to oven, bake for 20 minutes.

No Crust Quiche

Mix all ingredients until well blended

    8 eggs

    6 asparagus spears, cut into 1/2 inch pieces

    1/2 cup cottage cheese

    1/2 cup grated cheese

    1/4 cup onion, diced

    1 Tbsp Dijon mustard

Pour into pie pan. Bake at 350° for 40 to 45 minutes until center is puffy and top is golden brown.

Muffin-cup Quiche

Sauté 2 Tbsp butter

      1/2 onion, diced

Stir until onion is translucent. Then add

      10 ounces broccoli florets

      1/4 tsp salt

      1/4 cup water

Cook until broccoli is tender and water evaporates. Whisk together in medium bowl

      6 large eggs

      1 cup milk

      pinch of nutmeg

      1/8 tsp cayenne pepper (optional)

Put 1 scoop of broccoli/onion mix in each muffin cup. Sprinkle with cheese. Pour egg mixture over cheese. Bake at 350° for 40 minutes. Top with sour cream if desired.

Spinach Frittata

Same as Artichoke Frittata, but in place of artichoke hearts add 1 cup fresh spinach.

FISH

Broiled Mahi-Mahi or other fish fillets

Combine to make sauce:

    1/3 cup olive oil

    1/3 cup sesame seeds

    1/4 cup lemon juice

    salt and pepper to taste.

Baste 1 lb Mahi Mahi with sauce

Broil 8 to 10 minutes. Turn and baste again. Broil additional 8 minutes until flaky.

Fish fillets

Drench 2 fish fillets 3/8 inch thick with

    1-1/4 cup flour

    salt, pepper

Place in frying pan and sauté in butter about 3 minutes on each side. Sprinkle with

    1 1/2 tsp chopped parley

    1 Tbsp olive oil

Brown 2 Tbsp butter and combine with

    2 tsp lemon juice

Drizzle over fish.

Fish Fillet Amandine

Preheat oven to 400°

Combine

> 1 Tbsp mayonnaise
>
> 1 Tbsp Dijon mustard

Arrange on a greased cookie sheet

> 4 fillets (flounder or cod are good)
>
> 1/4 cup slivered almonds

Spread mayo mix evenly on each fillet. Sprinkle with almonds. Bake 10 to 12 minutes until fish flakes easily with a fork.

> (Good served with with Garlic Spinach)

Foil Dinner Fish

Place in the center of a piece of foil

> 1 fish fillet
>
> 1 cup sliced vegetables (carrots or asparagus or green beans or potatoes, etc.)

Drench with

> 1/2 cube butter melted
>
> 1/4 cup lemon juice
>
> 1/2 tsp garlic salt
>
> 1 handful cilantro, chopped

Fold foil over fish and veggies and close securely on top and sides. Bake in oven for 20 minutes at 400° or until veggies are tender.

Skillet Scallops

Melt in large skillet

 1/4 cup butter in large skillet.

Add   2 pounds scallops, fresh or frozen

Cook, stirring occasionally for 3 to 4 minutes

 1 package frozen pea pods

 2 tomatoes cut in eighths

Combine

 1/4 cup water

 2 Tbsp cornstarch

 1 Tbsp soy sauce

 1/2 tsp salt, 1/8 tsp pepper

Add to scallop mixture. Stir until thickened.

Serve over brown rice.

Salmon with Spinach

Sauté 1/2 onion

 1 Tbsp grated ginger

 4 salmon filets

Add to pan and bring to a simmer

 1 cup coconut milk

 2 handfuls fresh spinach

 Salt and pepper to taste

Simmer until coconut milk is reduced, serve over rice.

Tuna in Cheesy Rice

Bring to a boil and then simmer for 20-30 minutes until tender and water is absorbed

　　1 cup brown rice

　　2 1/4 cups water

In separate saucepan sauté

　　1/2 cube butter

　　1/2 cup chopped celery

　　1/3 cup chopped onion

Stir in

　　1-1/2 cup milk

　　1/2 tsp salt

　　1 cup shredded cheese

　　1 can albacore tuna

Pour sauce over cooked rice, stir in. Sauce will be liquid. Let sit to thicken.

LEGUMES

Black Beans and Rice
In soup pan bring to a boil and simmer until beans are tender

>1 cup dry black beans
>
>4 cups water

Add   1 onion, chopped

>2 bell peppers, chopped
>
>2 clove garlic
>
>1 bay leaf
>
>1 1/2 tsp salt
>
>1/4 tsp pepper

Add more water if needed and simmer for 2 1/2 hours.

Remove from heat, stir in 2 cups cooked brown rice. Serve.

Black Beans with Corn and Tomatoes
Combine

>2 cups cooked black beans
>
>1 cup corn, fresh or frozen
>
>1 cup tomatoes, diced
>
>1 clove garlic

Add   1 tsp parsley

>1/4 tsp red pepper flakes

Season with salt, pepper. Heat, add salsa to taste.

No-meat Chimichangas

Sauté in olive oil

>2 onions, chopped

>2 cloves garlic, chopped

Add, stir together, and heat to simmering

>3 cups cooked beans

>1 can chopped green chilies

>2 tsp oregano

>1 tsp salt

>½ tsp black pepper

>½ tsp crushed red pepper

>2 tsp dry cilantro or ¼ cup fresh cilantro

Spoon bean mixture onto tortillas, fold and deep-fry in olive or coconut oil. Serve with chopped lettuce, cabbage, tomatoes, grated cheese, guacamole, and sour cream.

Refried Bean Soup

Chop and sauté in olive oil

>1 cup celery, chopped

>1 onion, chopped

>1/2 bell pepper, chopped

>2 tsp oregano

>1 tsp salt

Add and bring to a simmer for 20 minutes

>4 cups vegetable broth

>4 cups refried beans

Season with salt and pepper to taste. Add salsa.

Katie's Chili Beans

Sauté in olive oil

       2 onions, diced

       2 bell peppers, diced

       4 celery stalks, diced

Add   8 cups cooked pinto or kidney beans

       6 oz tomato paste

       2 cups tomato sauce

       1 cup vegetable broth

       2 Tbsp chili powder

       2 tsp salt

       2 tsp cumin

       1 tsp oregano

       1 Tbsp dry cilantro or coriander

Add salsa and hot peppers to taste. Bring to a boil, simmer for an hour to blend flavors.

SALADS

Artichoke Avocado Salad
Place in flat bowl

> 1/2 head romaine lettuce, washed and chopped

Arrange on lettuce

> 4 hard cooked eggs, quartered
>
> 1-1/2 avocados, sliced
>
> 2 oranges, sectioned
>
> 1/2 jar marinated artichokes

Dressing:

Blend together

> 1/2 jar artichokes
>
> 2 Tbsp marinade
>
> 1 Tbsp olive oil
>
> 1 Tbsp red wine vinegar
>
> 1/2 avocado, peeled
>
> 1/2 cup plain yogurt
>
> 1/4 cup green onions, diced

Stir in and pour over salad or serve on side.

Beet and Potato Salad
Combine

> 1 cup cooked beets, diced
>
> 1 cup cooked, peeled potatoes, diced
>
> 1/2 cup apple, diced
>
> 1 bell pepper, diced
>
> 1 stalk celery, sliced

Toss in buttermilk type dressing.

Bean Salad

Toss   3 cups cooked beans

        1/4 cup green onions, minced

        1 clove garlic, minced

Add   2 to 3 Tbsp olive oil

        1/2 tsp oregano

        1/2 tsp thyme

        1/2 tsp sage

        salt and pepper

Let stand for 30 minutes Serve over greens with hard boiled eggs or tuna (optional).

Broccoli-Apple Salad

Combine

        2 large broccoli segments,

        1 apple, chopped

        1/4 red onion sliced

        1/2 cup walnuts or pecans

        1/2 cup raisins

Combine and fold over veggies

        1/2 cup mayonnaise

        1/2 cup sour cream

        2 Tbsp lemon juice

        1/4 tsp salt

Cabbage Salad

Brown in 350° oven

 1/2 cup slivered almonds

 2 Tbsp sesame seeds

Mix together

 1/2 head cabbage, chopped

 2 green onions, diced

Dressing:

 1/3 cup olive oil

 2 Tbsp vinegar

 1 tsp salt

 1/4 tsp pepper

Shake dressing well and pour over salad. Add nuts and seeds. Mix until all ingredients are well-coated.

Chopped Salad

Slice and chop

 1 head lettuce

 1/2 cabbage

 1/2 red cabbage

 1 bunch kale

 5 carrots, grated

 1 bunch spinach

 1 bunch arugula

Combine all greens in large bowl and toss together. Package in 1-gallon zip lock bags and use daily. Add cucumbers, tomatoes, avocadoes etc. (optional)

Cucumber Salad

Sprinkle with salt and let stand for 15 minutes on paper towel. Rinse and blot:

> 2 cucumbers, diced
>
> 1 tsp salt

Add and mix together

> 1/2 bell pepper, diced
>
> 2 green onions, sliced
>
> 1/2 cup plain yogurt
>
> 2 Tbsp lemon juice
>
> 1 Tbsp olive oil
>
> 1 clove garlic, minced
>
> 2 Tbsp fresh mint or 1/2 tsp dry mint

Cover and chill for 30 minutes. Serve over greens.

Fruit Salad

Combine

> 2 Tbsp honey
>
> 1 Tbsp lemon juice
>
> 1 cup plain yogurt
>
> 1/2 cup coconut flakes

Cut up a variety of fresh fruit. Fold yogurt dressing into fresh fruit and coconut

Chilean Onion and Tomato Salad

Slice 3 tomatoes and 1 onion

Drizzle with olive oil, salt to taste

Chill and serve

Papaya-Avocado Salad

Peel, seed and slice

 2 ripe papayas

 1 cup jicama

 2 ripe avocados

Mix together

 1/2 cup orange juice

 1/4 cup lime juice

 1 tsp rice vinegar

 1/4 tsp salt

Arrange papaya and avocado slices on a plate. Top with jicama. Drizzle with sour orange dressing

Rice Salad

In saucepan combine

> 1-1/2 cups brown rice

> 1/2 tsp salt

> 3 cups water

Bring to boil, cover and simmer about 25 minutes, until rice is tender, allow rice to cool.

Dressing:

In separate bowl whisk until well-blended

> 1/2 cup red wine vinegar

> 1 clove garlic, minced

> 1/3 cup olive oil

Add   salt and pepper

> 3 Tbsp parsley, chopped

> 3 Tbsp chives, chopped

Spoon rice into large bowl. Coat with vinegar dressing. Stir in 12 oz green beans, blanched for 2 minutes

> 12 oz cherry tomatoes, halved

> 2 cans tuna, drained

Bill's Tabouli Salad

Pour 2 cups boiling water over
       2/3 cup wheat

Cover and let stand 1 hour until wheat is light and fluffy.
Drain excess water.

Add   1/3 c onion, chopped
       2 tomatoes, diced
       3/4 cup fresh parsley, chopped
       2 Tbsp lemon juice
       1 Tbsp olive oil
       garlic powder
       1/4 cup red wine vinegar

Toss, chill for 1 hour. Serve over greens.

Tuna, Tomato, and Cucumber Salad

In large bowl combine
       1 cup grape tomatoes, halved
       1 cup cucumber, sliced
       1/2 red onion, sliced thin
       1/2 cup feta cheese
       1 can tuna, drained

Toss with Garlic Oil. Serve.

SAUCES, SALSAS, DRESSINGS

Artichoke Salsa

Drain and chop

     1 jar artichoke hearts

Add   1/4 cup olives

     2 Tbsp red onion, chopped

     3 tomatoes, diced

     1 clove garlic, diced

     2 Tbsp fresh basil, diced or 1 tsp dry basil

     salt and pepper

Cheese Sauce

Melt butter and combine with other ingredients in a skillet

     4 Tbsp butter

     2 Tbsp flour

     2 cups milk

     1/2 tsp salt

Stir until somewhat thickened then add

     2 cups grated cheese

     1/4 cup Parmesan cheese

Stir until blended. Pour over cooked vegetables or pasta, or use as a cheese dip. Also great for macaroni and cheese!

Chilies con Queso Salsa

Sauté in olive oil

> 1 onion, diced

Add and simmer for 5 minutes

> 1 can chopped green chilies

> 1 can stewed tomatoes

Stir in 1/4 tsp baking soda

> 16 ounces grated cheese

Thin with up to 1/2 cup milk if needed.

Easy Mayonnaise

> 1 whole egg

> 1/2 tsp salt

> 1/2 tsp dried mustard

> 2 tsp lemon juice

> 1 Tbsp white wine vinegar

> 1 cup olive oil

Combine all ingredients except olive oil in blender. While blending on medium speed add olive oil very slowly until emulsified.

Pesto Mayonnaise

Combine 1/2 cup Easy Mayonnaise

> 2 tsp mustard

> 1 Tbsp dry basil

> 1/2 Tbsp garlic powder

> 1 Tbsp Parmesan cheese

> Salt and pepper to taste

Use in place of plain mayo.

Garlic Oil

Combine in saucepan

> 1/2 cup olive oil
> 3 cloves garlic, chopped
> 1/4 tsp red pepper flakes
> salt, pepper to taste

Simmer on low for 10 minutes. Remove from heat and chill for 15 minutes. Keep at room temperature.

Guacamole

Cut and mash 5 ripe avocados

Stir in

> 1/2 cup sour cream
> 1/3 cup sweet onion, chopped
> 2 tomatoes chopped
> 1/4 cup fresh cilantro, chopped
> garlic salt
> 2 tsp lime juice

Pico de Gallo

Chop and combine:

> 2-3 medium tomatoes
> ½ medium onion
> 1 green pepper
> ½ c cilantro
> 1 lime juiced
> 1 tsp salt

Let sit for about ten minutes. Serve fresh

Spinach Dip

Sauté in butter about 3 minutes

      1/4 onion, diced

      2 cloves garlic, diced

Add   1 Tbsp flour

      1-3/4 cup cream

Stir until thickened, about 2 minutes.

Add   18 oz fresh or frozen spinach, chopped

      1 can water chestnuts, drained

      1 cup shredded cheese

      salt and pepper to taste

Spoon into casserole. Sprinkle with 1/4 cup Parmesan cheese. Bake at 425° for 10-15 minutes.

Terrific Tomato Sauce

Combine in pressure cooker

      2 Tbsp olive oil

      6 cloves garlic

      1 onion, chopped

      5 pounds tomatoes, diced (about 10 or 12)

      1 Tbsp salt

      1/2 Tbsp black pepper

      1-1/2 Tbsp Italian seasoning

      1/4 tsp crushed red pepper

      1 bay leaf

      1-1/2 tsp basil

Pressure cook for 10 minutes. Allow pressure to drop before opening. Makes about 4 quarts. Perfect for spaghetti.

Vinaigrette

Combine 3/4 cup olive oil

     1/4 cup vinegar

     1 green onion, minced

     2 Tbsp basil pesto

     1/2 tsp garlic powder

     salt and pepper to taste

     1/2 to 3/4 cups water

Shake well to blend and pour over salad.

White Sauce

Melt 2 Tbsp butter and combine with

     2 Tbsp flour

     1/2 tsp salt

     1/4 tsp pepper

     1/2 tsp onion salt

     1/2 cup milk

     1/2 cup sour cream

Stir until thickened. *Don't overheat*. Good over green beans, broccoli and other vegetables.

SIDE DISHES

Garlic Spinach
Sauté in olive oil
    2 cups mushrooms
Add and cook until wilted
    1 bag baby spinach (5 ounces)
    1 cup cherry tomatoes, halved
    Garlic salt to taste

Herbed New Potatoes
    12 small new potatoes
Peel a 1/2-inch strip around the middle of each potato and place in saucepan filled with cold water covering potatoes by 2 inches. Bring to boil for about 20 minutes or until potatoes can be easily pierced by a fork. Drain.
Melt and combine
    2 Tbsp butter
    2 Tbsp fresh parsley or 1-1/2 tsp dry parsley
    2 Tbsp fresh minced chives or 1-1/2 tsp dry chives
Drizzle over potatoes. Toss to coat.

Mexican Brown Rice

In a hot skillet toast 2 cups dry brown rice

Combine, bring to a boil, and pour over rice

  2 cups water or vegetable broth

  1 can tomato puree

  2 onions, diced

  1 clove garlic, diced

  1 Tbsp parsley or cilantro, chopped

Cover and cook on low for about 40 minutes.

Ratatouille

Steam for 2 minutes

  2 cups broccoli florets

  1 cup cauliflower bits

Sauté in 2 Tbsp oil for 3 minutes

  1 red onion, wedged

  1 clove garlic, chopped

Add steamed veggies to skillet. Stir-fry 2 minutes.

Add   2 Tbsp teriyaki sauce

  1 tsp lemon pepper

  1 yellow squash, sliced

  1 zucchini, sliced

  2 tomatoes, wedged

Stir-fry another couple of minutes. Turn into casserole

Sprinkle with

  1/2 cup Parmesan cheese

  2 Tbsp sesame seeds

 Broil for 3 to 5 minutes until toasted

.

Sliced Baked Potatoes

Slice: 4 large potatoes in ¼ inch slices

Place slices overlapping in buttered 13 x 9 inch dish. Mix

    1⁄4 cup olive oil

    1⁄4 cup melted butter

Brush slices liberally. Top with

    2 cloves garlic minced

    1 tsp salt

    1⁄2 tsp dry thyme

Bake at 400° for 25 to 30 minutes

Stuffed potatoes

Simmer: I onion diced

Cool onion in a bowl.

Scoop out 2 baked potatoes and add to onion.

Stir in 1⁄2 cup cottage cheese

    1⁄2 cup buttermilk

    1⁄4 cup Parmesan cheese

Mound mixture back into potato skins. Sprinkle with green onion.

Zucchini and Tomatoes

Melt and sauté:

    3 Tbsp butter

    1 lb zucchini, sliced

    1/4 cup green onion, chopped

Add   2 cups tomatoes, diced

    1 tsp dry tarragon

    1/2 tsp salt, pepper

Cook five minutes over medium heat.

Zucchini au Gratin

Peel, cook and drain

    8 small zucchini, sliced lengthwise

Lay side by side in casserole. Drizzle with oil.

Mix together and sprinkle over zucchini

    2 Tbsp parsley, chopped

    1/2 tsp oregano

    salt and pepper

    1 cup dry bread crumbs

    1/2 cup Parmesan cheese

Bake at 350° for 20 minutes.

SOUPS and STEWS

Acorn Squash Soup
Pressure cook about 4 minutes
>2 acorn squash, halved

Sauté and stir in with cooked, peeled squash
>1 onion, chopped

>1 carrot, chopped

>1 clove garlic, chopped

Add   3 1/2 cups broth

Simmer 20 minutes, puree.

Add   1/2 tsp nutmeg
>1/2 tsp cinnamon

>1 cup milk

Bring to a simmer. Serve.

Black Bean Soup
Sauté in olive oil
>1 onion, chopped

>3 cloves garlic, chopped

>1 tsp cumin

>1 tsp chili powder

>1/2 tsp oregano

>1 bay leaf

>1/4 tsp red pepper flakes

Add   6 cups cooked black beans with liquid
>2 tsp salt

Simmer 15 minutes, add black pepper and cilantro to taste.

Chunky Potato Soup

Bring 4 cups of water to boil in a saucepan.

Add 6 medium red potatoes, peeled and cubed

Cook until tender, drain and set aside liquid and potatoes.

Sauté in 3 Tbsp olive oil or butter

      1 onion, diced

Add 3 Tbsp flour

      1/4 tsp crushed red pepper

      Salt and pepper

Stir 3 or 4 minutes until thickened.

Gradually add potatoes

      1 cup drained liquid from potatoes

      3 cups milk

      1 cup shredded cheese

Simmer for 30 minutes stirring as needed.

Corn Chowder

Sauté 1 onion, diced

Add   3 cups vegetable broth

      6 potatoes, diced

Boil gently until potatoes are tender

Add   2 cups fresh or frozen corn

      2 Tbsp flour

      3 Tbsp butter

      3 cups milk

      3/4 cup grated cheese

Stir until thickened. If desired add one can chopped green chilies

Portuguese Cabbage Soup

Combine in soup pot and simmer for 1 hour

      10 cups water or vegetable broth

      1 cup dry kidney beans

      1 onion, chopped

      1/2 cup cabbage, chopped

      1 Tbsp vinegar

      1 Tbsp salt, pepper

Add and simmer for about 45 minutes

      1 pound kale, chopped

Add and simmer until potatoes are tender

      1 cup water

      2 cups potatoes, cubed

Serve.

Lentil-Vegetable Soup

In casserole dish brown in 2 Tbsp olive oil

      4 potatoes, cubed

      3 onions, chopped

      1/2 pound mushrooms, sliced

      1 clove garlic, diced

Add and sauté briefly

      1-1/2 cups carrots, sliced

      1 cup celery, chopped

Add remaining ingredients and simmer for about an hour

      1-1/2 cups dry lentils

      1-1/2 cups tomatoes, chopped

      5 cups water or broth

      2 bay leaves

1 tsp dry basil

3 Tbsp soy sauce

1 Tbsp Worcestershire sauce

Sprinkle with parsley and serve.

Minestrone

Sauté 1 onion, chopped

    1 clove garlic, diced

    1 leek, diced

Combine in large kettle with sautéed vegetables and simmer for 20 minutes

    6 cups Vegetable Broth

    4 cups cooked kidney beans

    6 tomatoes, chopped

    2 cups cabbage, shredded

    2 potatoes, diced

    2 carrots, diced

    2 stalks celery, chopped

Add and simmer an additional 10 minutes until macaroni is tender

Add   2 Tbsp minced parsley

    1/2 tsp thyme

    1/2 tsp oregano

    1/4 cup tomato paste

    2 zucchini, diced

    1 cup elbow macaroni (look for whole wheat pasta)

Simmer, sprinkle with Parmesan cheese and serve.

Potato Green Chili Soup

Sauté 1 onion, chopped
      2 cloves garlic, chopped
      4 to 6 potatoes, cubed
Stir in
      2 Tbsp flour
      4 cups vegetable broth
Bring to boil and simmer 10 to 15 minutes.
Add   1 cup milk
      1 can green chilies
Simmer 10 minutes or until potatoes are tender. Add salt and pepper to taste.

Pumpkin Soup

Combine 4 cups vegetable broth
      1-1/2 tsp salt
      3 cups pumpkin, cooked and pureed
      1 onion, chopped
      1/2 tsp thyme
      1 clove garlic, chopped
Bring to boil, simmer for 30 minutes. Puree, reheat, Add
      1 cup milk
      1 tsp dry parsley or cilantro or
      add fresh parsley or cilantro

Sonora Bean Soup

Pressure cook in 6 cups water for 15 minutes

     1 cup dry pinto beans

     1/2 onion, chopped

     1 clove garlic, chopped

     2 Tbsp olive oil

Mash or puree beans.

Add   1-1/2 cup grated cheese

     6 green onions, minced

     Salsa to taste.

Split Pea Soup

Combine

     1 16 oz package green split peas

     2 quarts water

     2 stalks celery, chopped

     1 onion, chopped

     1 carrot, chopped

     1/2 tsp black pepper

     1/4 tsp red pepper flakes

     1 bay leaf

     1 clove garlic

     salt

Bring to boil, cover and simmer for 1 hour. Puree if desired.

Vegetable Stew

Sauté in 2 Tbsp olive oil

      1 onion, chopped

Add   1/2 cup Terrific Tomato Sauce

      2 Tbsp balsamic vinegar

      2 cups vegetable broth

      2 pounds potatoes, cubed

      1 pound carrots, chopped

      3 celery stalks, chopped

      2 cloves garlic, chopped

      salt and pepper

Bring to a boil, simmer for 35 minutes until tender.

Vegetable Broth

Sauté in 1/4 cup olive oil

      4 onions, chopped

      4 carrots, diced

      4 celery stalks with leaves

      4 parsnips, diced

Add   3 cups water

      1 Tbsp salt

Add seasonings in a cheesecloth bag:

      1/3 c dry parsley

      2 tsp peppercorns

      2 bay leaves

      1/2 tsp basil

      1/2 tsp thyme

Bring to boil. Cover and simmer for 3 hours. Strain broth.
Makes 8 to 12 cups

Fresh Vegetable Soup

Combine and bring to a boil

    4 cups water

    2 potatoes, cubed

    2 carrots, sliced

    1 zucchini, sliced

    1 onion, diced

    1 cup celery, sliced

    1/2 c celery leaves, chopped

    1 tsp salt

Cover and simmer for 20 minutes until carrots and potatoes are tender.

Add   2 cups spinach

      1/2 tsp pepper

Cover and simmer for 2 more minutes.

Tomato-Basil Soup

Combine 2 cups Terrific Tomato Sauce with 1 cup milk Heat and serve.

VEGETARIAN ENTRES

Fresh vegetables, raw or cooked, are always good.

Brazilian Empanadas
Filling:
Sauté 1 onion, diced
      1 clove garlic
Add and simmer 20 minutes
      1/2 tsp coriander
      pinch ginger
      2 tomatoes, chopped
      2 Tbsp parsley
      1/3 cup chopped green olives
      2 cups black beans
      salt, pepper
Pastry:
Combine
      2-3/4 cups flour
      1/2 tsp salt
Cut in
      2/3 cup olive or coconut oil
Add   2 egg yolks beaten in 1 cup water
Drizzle egg water over pastry flour tossing with a fork until mixture holds together. Form a ball and roll dough 1/2 inch thick. Cut in circles, place 1/3 cup filling on each circle. Fold and pinch closed forming half-circle. Bake at 375° for 25 to 35 minutes.

Broccoli Casserole

Cut into one inch pieces and cook

>   4 cups fresh or frozen broccoli

Combine with the broccoli

>   1-1/2 cups celery stalks, sliced
>
>   3/4 cup mushrooms, sliced

In separate bowl mix together

>   3/4 cup milk
>
>   1 cup sour cream
>
>   1-1/2 tsp salt,
>
>   1/4 tsp pepper

Pour liquid ingredients over vegetables and turn into a greased casserole dish. Sprinkle with

>   1/4 cup grated cheese
>
>   Dot with butter

Bake at 350° for 20 to 25 minutes.

Broccoli, Potato, Mushroom Sauté

Boil for about 10 minutes

>   5 potatoes sliced

Sauté 1 onion sliced

>   ½ cup mushrooms, sliced

Add   16 oz bag frozen broccoli

>   Potato slices
>
>   Salt and pepper

Stir together and continue cooking until all vegetables are tender.

Broccoli Empanadas

Prepare 1 loaf Basic Bread Dough.

Microwave

      2 cups chopped broccoli

Sauté 1 clove garlic in olive oil

Add cooked broccoli. Cook for about 3 minutes. Remove from heat and mix in

      1 cup shredded cheese

      1/2 cup Parmesan cheese

      2 roasted red peppers, chopped

      1 tsp oregano

      1/2 tsp salt

      1/4 tsp black pepper

Divide bread dough into 8 pieces. Roll out into 6 inch circles. Spoon 1/8 of broccoli mixture onto each circle. Fold dough over to form half circle. Press edges with a fork to seal. Prick holes in empanada top. Place on baking sheets. Bake at 375° about 25 minutes.

Brown Rice with Veggies

In skillet sauté in oil

      1 cup pecan or walnut halves

Set aside.

Add oil to skillet and sauté

      1 cup broccoli florets

      1 bell pepper sliced

Add and stir in

      1 zucchini, sliced

      1 yellow squash, sliced

Add   1 cup snow pea pods

      1/4 cup water

Cover and cook 1-2 minutes until vegetables are tender.

In a large bowl toss

      3 cups hot brown rice

      3 Tbsp parsley.

Top with veggies and toasted nuts

Calzone

Prepare Basic Bread Dough, enough for 2 loaves. Set aside.
Sauté in olive oil

> 1 pound mushrooms, chopped
>
> 6 ounces chopped black olives
>
> 1 onion, diced
>
> 1 zucchini, chopped
>
> 1 bell pepper, chopped
>
> 2 cloves garlic, chopped
>
> Salt and pepper to taste

Drain well and blot dry. Divide into four portions. Roll out half a loaf of bread dough fairly thin (1/4 of total dough) Pile vegetables on one side of flat rolled dough covering about a third of the surface.
Pour 1/2 cup of Terrific Tomato Sauce over vegetables.
Sprinkle each calzone with

> Parmesan cheese
>
> 1/2 cup mozzarella cheese

Add   cooked crab (optional)
Dampen edges of dough, starting at side without filling, pull the dough and fold over. Pinch closed along side.
Make 3 vent holes for steam to escape. Bake at 420° for 10 minutes. Lower temperature to 350° and continue cooking for 20 minutes.

Cheese and Spinach Manicotti

Cook 8 manicotti shells as directed on package. Combine

> 2 cups cottage cheese
>
> 1 - 3 oz. pkg. cream cheese, softened
>
> 1/4 cup Parmesan cheese
>
> 1/4 cup parsley, chopped
>
> 1 egg, slightly beaten
>
> 1/4 tsp salt

Stuff shells with cheese mixture. Smother with 2 cups Terrific Tomato Sauce, 1/4 cup Parmesan cheese.

Bake at 350° for 25 to 30 minutes.

Steam 10 oz. spinach, fresh or frozen. Drain well and spoon down center of manicotti. Garnish with parsley.

Cheesy Enchiladas

Sauce:

Heat and stir in 2 Tbsp olive oil

> 1 Tbsp flour
>
> 3 Tbsp chili powder

Add   1-1/2 cup vegetable broth

> 1-1/2 cup tomato sauce
>
> 1/2 tsp cumin

Pour half the sauce into a casserole dish. Fry tortillas in hot oil and place in pan with sauce. Fill each tortilla with grated cheese and cooked beans and roll up, filling pan. Pour remaining sauce over filled tortillas. Sprinkle liberally with cheese. Bake 20 mins at 350°

Mexican Lasagna

Sauce:

Sauté 1 onion, diced

       2 stalks celery chopped

       1 bell pepper, chopped

       1 clove garlic

Add and simmer

       3 cups tomato sauce

       4 tomatoes, diced

       3/4 cup water

       1/2 cup salsa

Add   2 cups mushrooms, sliced

Filling:

Mix together

       2 cups cooked pinto beans

       1 cup onion, chopped

       1 clove garlic

       1 can chopped green chilies

       1/2 tsp oregano

       3 tomatoes, diced

Layer tortillas and filling, sprinkle with cheese, pour 1/4 cup sauce over each layer. Repeat, add additional cheese on top. Bake at 400° for 5 minutes. Garnish with lettuce, olives, etc.

Potato and Apple Casserole

In saucepan cook until tender

    2 Tbsp butter

    3/4 c shredded apple

Stir in 2 Tbsp flour

    1/4 tsp pepper

Add and bring to a boil while stirring

    1/2 cup vegetable broth

    1/2 cup milk

Turn off heat and stir in

    3/4 cup cheese, shredded

Layer in oiled casserole dish

    1 pound baking potatoes, thinly sliced

Cover 1/2 the potatoes with 1/2 the prepared sauce. Repeat layer of potatoes and sauce. Bake at 350° covered for 40 minutes. Uncover, continue baking for 30 minutes until potatoes are tender.

Stew

Dice and sauté 1 onion in 2 Tbsp olive oil

Stir in 2 cups vegetable broth

    1/2 cup tomato sauce

    2 Tbsp balsamic vinegar

    2 lb potatoes

    1 lb carrots

    3 celery stalks

    Other vegetables as desired

    Salt, pepper and garlic to taste

Simmer until vegetables are tender.

Stuffed Grape Leaves

Filling:

Sauté 2 onions, minced

Add and bring to a boil

      1 1/2 cups dry brown rice

      3 cups water

Add remaining ingredients

      2 Tbsp currants or raisins

      1 Tbsp cinnamon

      1 tsp allspice

      1 tsp olive oil

      2 cups cooked beans

      2 Tbsp salt

      1 Tbsp pepper

      1 tsp oregano

      1 Tbsp dry mint

      1 Tbsp dry parsley

Wrap in grape leaves, bake at 375° until tender.

Succotash

Sauté in olive oil

      1 onion, chopped

      1 bell pepper, diced

      6 potatoes, cubed

      2 tomatoes, diced

Add   2 cups frozen corn

      2 cups cooked beans, pinto or lima

      2 cups water

Bring to boil, simmer 20 minutes or until water is absorbed.

Vegetable Stir Fry

Chop all vegetables and stir-fry in hot oil

      2 celery stalks

      1 green pepper

      3 carrots

      1 onion

      1 cup cabbage

      1 can water chestnuts

      1 cup or can mushrooms

Stir until tender.

Add

      1/2 cup water

      1/4 cup soy sauce

      1/8 cup corn starch

Stir until thickened. Serve over brown rice

Yams and Carrot Casserole

Preheat oven to 400°.

In large bowl combine

   2 large sweet potatoes, sliced thin

   8 medium carrots, sliced

   1 large onion, diced

   2 cloves garlic, chopped

In a separate bowl whisk together

   Juice of 1 orange

   3 Tbsp butter+ 2 Tbsp olive oil

   1 tsp salt

   1 tsp sweet paprika

   1/2 tsp ground cumin

   1/2 tsp ground ginger

   1/4 tsp cinnamon

   1/4 tsp black pepper

   pinch of cayenne pepper

Pour over vegetables, toss to coat. Bake in roasting pan about 35 minutes.

Food Substitutions

1 Tbs cornstarch		2 Tbs white flour
1 cup sugar		2/3 cup honey
1 cup sugar		½ cup maple syrup
1 tsp arrowroot		1 Tbs white flour
1 cup bread crumbs		1 cup ground oats
1 tsp cream of tartar		2 tsp lemon juice
1 tsp powdered ginger		2 tsp fresh
1 Tbs fresh herbs		1 tsp dry
1 cup mayonnaise		1 cup plain yogurt
¼ cup fresh mint		1 Tbs dry

Food equivalents

1 pound yams		3 medium
3 medium apples		3 cups sliced
3 medium bananas		1 1/3 cup mashed
1 pound bread		15-20 slices
1 pound flour		3 ½ - 4 cups
Dash		2-3 drops
1 Tbs		3 tsp
4 Tbs		¼ cup
1/3 cup		4 Tbs + 1 tsp
1 pint		2 cups or 16 oz
1 quart		4 cups
1 gallon		4 quarts
1 pound		16 ounces
1 ounce		2 Tablespoons
1 ounce		28.4 grams
1 kilogram		2.2 pounds

1 cup dry rice		3 cups cooked
1 cup cream		2 cups whipped
1 cup egg white		8-10 eggs
1 cup egg yolk		12-14 eggs
1 gelatin packet		1 Tbs gelatin
1 medium lemon		3 Tbs juice
1 medium lime		2 Tbs juice
12 oz evaporated milk		1 2/3 cups
1 large onion		1 cup chopped
1 medium orange		½ cup juice
1 pint berries		1 ¾ cups
1 slice bread		½ cup crumbs
1 bouillon cube		1 cup broth
1 cube butter		½ cup
¼ pound cheese		1 cup shredded
8 oz cheese		2 cups shredded
8 oz cottage cheese		1 cup
3 oz cream cheese		6 Tbs
1 square chocolate		1 oz
1 pound walnuts		2 ¾ cups
3 medium potatoes		1 pound
3 medium potatoes		2 ¼ cups
1 pound raisins		3 cups
1 pound oil		2 cups

Step 1	M	T	W	Th	F	S	Su
Greens							
Fruit							
Step 2							
Fish							
Step 3							
Breads							
Cereal							
Step 4							
Vines							
Roots							
Legumes							
Step 5							
No process							
Step 6							
Eggs							
Dairy							
Step 7							
Healthy oil							
Honey							
Nuts spice							
Step 8							
Water							
Step 9							
Exercise							

Use the check-list chart to make multiple copies and track your progress. .

REFERENCES

1 Hyman, Mark, *The Blood Sugar Solution*, Little, Brown Spark; 28 Feb 2012

2 Kimball, Edward L. *The History of LDS Temple Admission Standards* p 159. 1998.

3 *Journal of Discourses*, Vol. 9, p 35.

4 *Doctrine and Covenants Church History, Seminary Teacher Manual*, Church of Jesus Christ of Latter-Day Saints.

5 *Minutes of first Presidency and Council Meeting, Journal History of the Church of Jesus Christ of Latter-Day Saints*, LDS Archives, May 5, 1898.

6 Alexander, Thomas G. *The Word of Wisdom: From Principle to Requirement*, Dialogue: A journal of Mormon Thought. p 179.

7 Smith, Joseph F., *Conference Reports,* p 14. October 1914.

8 Clark, James R. *Messages of the First Presidency*. Vol 5, p 163.

9 Bikman, Benjamin. *The Plagues of Prosperity*, speeches.byu.edu/talks, 2019.

10www.fairmormon.org/answers/Word_of_Wisdom
Eat_meat_sparingly

11 www.ncbi.nlm.nih.gov/pmc/articles/PMC5475232/
12Ioannides, John
https://journals.plos.org/plosmedicine/article?id=10.1
371/journal.pmed.0020124
13 www.drheatherpaulson.com/pescatarian-diet-
reduces-cancer-risk/
14www.ncbi.nlm.nih.gov/pmc/articles/PMC1182327/
15www.academic.oup.com/ajcn/article/97/1/127/457
6988
16 *Doctrine and Covenants Student Manual 2002*,
Church of Jesus Christ of Latter-Day Saints, p 14.
17 *Processed Food Facts*—Zest Moose.
https://thezestymoose.com/tag/processed-food-facts/
18 https://draxe.com/olive-oil-benefits/
19 McNamara, Robert K, Susan E Carlson. *Role of
Omega 3 Fatty Acids in Brain Development and
Function*, Department of Psychiatry, University of
Cincinnati School of Medicine. 2006.
20www.lifeextension.com/magazine/2008/1/report_d
hafishoil/page-
21www.ncbi.nlm.nih.gov/pmc/articles/PMC3046737/
22 https://chriskresser.com/how-too-much-omega-6-
and-not-enough- omega-3-is-making...
23 *Rethinking Restrictive Diets: Should We Be Eating
more Dairy and Carbs?* elmageGutReportgoop.com
24 www.ncbi.nlm.nih.gov/pmc/articles/PMC4808858/
25 www.ncbi.nlm.nih.gov/pmc/articles/PMC3046737/
26 Donin, Hayim Halevy, *To Be a Jew,* Basic Books,
August 6, 2008.

ABOUT THE AUTHOR

Karen Hopkins is a member of the Church of Jesus Christ of Latter-day Saints. Born in California, she attended Brigham Young University and received a degree from the College of Family Living in 1971. She returned to BYU and received a second degree in Spanish. Karen has lived and worked in a variety places including Central and South America, Europe, the Middle East and India. She has always been interested in health and nutrition and its impact on her family. Karen is the mother of nine children.